Same Sex Love, 1700–1957: A History and Research Guide

For Gill and Johnny, with all my love
Thank you for believing in me

Same Sex Love, 1700–1957: A History and Research Guide

By

GILL ROSSINI

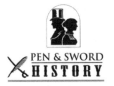

PEN & SWORD
HISTORY

First published in Great Britain in 2017 by
Pen & Sword History
an imprint of
Pen & Sword Books Ltd
47 Church Street
Barnsley
South Yorkshire
S70 2AS

Copyright © Gill Rossini, 2017

ISBN 978 1 47385 423 9

Printed and bound in Malta
By Gutenberg Press Ltd.

Pen & Sword Books Ltd incorporates the Imprints of Pen & Sword Books
Archaeology, Atlas, Aviation, Battleground, Discovery, Family History, History,
Maritime, Military, Naval, Politics, Railways, Select, Transport, True Crime,
Fiction, Frontline Books, Leo Cooper, Praetorian Press, Seaforth Publishing,
Wharncliffe and White Owl.

For a complete list of Pen & Sword titles please contact
PEN & SWORD BOOKS LIMITED
47 Church Street, Barnsley, South Yorkshire, S70 2AS, England
E-mail: enquiries@pen-and-sword.co.uk
Website: www.pen-and-sword.co.uk

Contents

Acknowledgements

The subject of this book has been a part of my life and, latterly, my teaching since I first discovered Radclyffe Hall in the 1980s, and so my thanks and gratitude must go back a very long way. I have drawn on so many archives, resources and fellow historians it would be hard to single any one out, and also rather unfair. So to all of you, I give my sincere thanks for your help and support.

More recently, this book would not now be available in print without the wonderful support of no less than three Pen and Sword editors. To Jen Boyle: thank you for believing in this project from the start and giving me the chance to prove myself as a trustworthy custodian of a sensitive subject with my history of adoption; without your initial faith in me this book would not have happened. To Eloise Hansen, who succeeded Jen at Pen and Sword, a huge thanks for taking up the same-sex proposal and guiding it towards a commission. Finally, to Heather Williams, my current editor, my enormous gratitude for your patience and understanding at a very difficult time for me personally, and for sticking with me; thank you also for your sage advice and guidance, and for being my professional rock. Also to Karyn Burnham, sincere thanks for your expert help with the draft, and for making it an altogether more professional piece of work.

To my students in Wales, Cheshire, and Lancashire, who have been the most wonderful, lively, inspiring, and erudite collective muse any historian could ever have: my deepest gratitude to you all for joining me on the fabulous journey that is the study of history. I have always told you all that we learn together and as a team, and so we have. I am honoured to have you as colleague historians.

And to my partner Gill, and my son Johnny; my unending thanks and love for allowing me to dream and for supporting me in my endeavours. Dreams have no value if you have no-one to share them with.

List of Illustrations

Introduction

The Purpose of This Book

This book is about the love of those who were attracted to their own gender, the challenges many of those people faced, and how they tried to live their lives within the constraints of the era and society into which they were born. Here, you will meet builders, soldiers, sailors, housewives, artists, mothers and fathers, drunkards, policemen, drivers, celebrities, shopkeepers, prostitutes, in fact, pretty much every type of person and job you can think of. They all, by and large, tried to go about their business like everyone else with one slight difference: they loved people of the same gender as their own. Many such stories are told here. You will meet people who lived in obscurity, and yet some names you will recognise; some even are household names, or were in their heyday. Other people were dragged from obscurity by their sexuality and became public property, if only for a brief moment. I have included a selection of better-known people to illustrate the point that there were a large number of male and female homosexuals who, being public figures, were lavished with respect and held in awe, but still rarely broadcast their same-sex loves to anyone other than their close circle. Everyone was affected by the repressive attitudes and laws of society, whoever they were.

Thankfully, bureaucracy – on the whole – treated most people in certain historical periods equally. No matter what your sexuality, you were expected to fill in your census form and become part of the census enumerator's returns. It was compulsory to have your birth, marriage, and death recorded, and to comply with all registration laws. You needed to work hard and stay out of the workhouse, and if you got into trouble or made a scene, you could expect to end up in the local newspaper. If you broke the law, you would be punished – although some people were punished more harshly because of their choice of partner.

Essentially, because many of the people in this narrative are pretty ordinary, they crop up in the same ways as anyone else in the records. However, sometimes people had cause to disguise their life in some way to maintain that veneer of respectability; this happened in all walks of life and all levels of society. Those in the establishment had to be an example to their 'inferiors'; and the working and middle classes were under great pressure to be 'respectable' and 'ordinary', and not to stand out as different.

Those who loved within their own gender were not the only minority group within society. The poor, the illegitimate, petty criminals, and the disabled, were all scorned and side-lined, deserted by family and community who were afraid of their difference, which at the time would have been seen as a sign of failure – even in a child (through their mother). What society and family did not recognise, of course, is that the line between 'normal' and 'different' is fine, if not diffuse, and that is perhaps why so many were actually frightened of associating with such minorities. They feared that they might be infected by the very difference that marked these people out.

This book aims to describe the diverse nature of same-sex relationships across a broad span of years, and to remind the reader that love between two people of the same gender can take many forms in spite of the many cultural, legal and societal restrictions faced by those who fell in love outside the norm of the day. Yet at the same time, as has been stated above, it is the story of many ordinary people. History demonstrates that the ordinary and extraordinary can, and should, live side by side.

Terminology

The vast majority of people today who are culturally aware will be familiar with what the words gay, lesbian or bisexual mean in what is an increasingly complex and nuanced spectrum of sexuality. Most will also know that 'LGB' are the collective initials for the abovementioned words and, because society uses them freely, many people recognise them and accept them, including those to whom these ' labels' fit as descriptors. However, the words and phrases used to describe individuals who have felt same-sex attraction over the centuries have varied enormously and the terms used today would have been unrecognisable to people 150 years ago ('lesbian' being the possible exception because of its classical origins).

INTRODUCTION

It would be false to use terms that are not contemporary to any given period in history to describe people we now refer to as gay, lesbian and bisexual, and every effort is made in this book to avoid such a collision of cultures. Labels bring with them mental images of what a person is like, can and cannot do, and of their lifestyle, that would be inappropriate for their time. If you addressed an eighteenth century man in a same-sex relationship as 'queer' or 'gay', he would not have the faintest idea what you meant by it! We cannot impose anachronistic words on people from history, so wherever necessary in the narrative, the historically appropriate terms are introduced, and references are kept contemporary to the period and/or as neutral as possible.

Where's the T?

This book is the story of individuals who felt same-sex attraction, and of the society they lived in and its reactions to them. However, anyone who reads it may wonder why it addresses only these groups and not any people who may now be regarded as transgendered or transsexual, whether via their self-identification or retrospectively by researchers and historians. There are two reasons why the 'T' has been left off the 'LGB'.

First, this book covers a wide span of dates and it is something of a juggling act to say everything I consider important in so small a space. To add the history of transgender as a separate subject to the narrative could make the story so superficial as to reduce its value as a research tool.

The second reason is one of respect. The complex, wonderful and colourful world of transgender history is relatively new – even more so than the history of homosexuality – and new research and commentaries are being released on a regular basis. The academics who research this field are, by and large, transgendered themselves and will have the innate understanding of, and empathy for their subject that hopefully, as a gay woman, I have for this book's subject matter. The intention is, therefore, to respectfully step aside from a detailed analysis of transgendered people in history and let more expert historians write of it, and to concentrate here on same-sex relationships only.

This is not to set rigid boundaries, however. Without the thoughts of the people involved (and this is especially difficult to ascertain if they did not leave a written record), it is impossible to say for sure whether, for example, a woman who cross-dressed and who also had a female partner was passing as male simply in order to support them both on a higher wage, or because she innately believed herself to be male and this was her way of expressing that innermost feeling. When telling the stories in this book of people who did cross-dress, assumptions about why they did so have been avoided unless there is a clear, verifiable reason for it.

The Ethics of Researching Same-sex Relationships in History

Not so long ago – and in some countries in the world today, this would still apply – to have your homosexuality broadcast in the mass media was a truly devastating event. Your relationships, career, and income would most probably all suffer; the damage to your peace of mind and to your family could be incalculable. Even rumours within a community, gossip, and innuendo could cause people to avoid you both socially and at work. One could find oneself exiled from family and friends.

In the past, however, many people successfully kept their relationships as discreet as possible throughout their lives, and passed into history without causing any ripples at all on the waters of time. Often their families colluded in this discretion or secrecy, never talking about certain events or people, shushing children if they asked too many questions and destroying evidence such as letters, diaries and photographs.

Everything has changed. We now live in a world where it is increasingly easy to conduct casual research on the internet using major history resources, all nicely indexed and collated for anyone, historian or otherwise, to delve into. Then there are the family historians, with their endless questions – I am an avid genealogist myself and have been since the 1970s. We want to know everything about our ancestors, where they lived, what jobs they had, who they lived with, what they looked like – no resource is left unexplored, and the more elusive a person is, the more we want to know about them. That mysterious uncle or aunt who never married but had a 'special friend' who sometimes came to tea, the unspoken stories and opinions that we try to piece together from what is left to us in documentary sources, the intriguing same-sex household that a relative lived in from one census return to the next, the articles in local newspapers about court cases that our ancestors hoped would never see the light of day again once they became the next day's kindling – all these and more are of intense interest to us. Moreover, since the huge growth in the popularity of social history, especially since

INTRODUCTION

the mid-twentieth century, the more trials and tribulations an ancestor had, the more they suffered and the more they tried to conceal, the more vigorously we pursue them. It is now almost a badge of honour for a genealogist to have a transgressor or two in one's family tree, be they criminal, immoral, destitute, antisocial or just plain desperate. Yet in the twenty-first century, most people think it is also very bad form to 'out' (reveal to the public) a living person's sexuality in the media – unless the informers are from the lower end of the tabloid press, or online gossip columns. The question is this: how ethical is it to unearth these stories when the people involved in historical events tried so hard – often at great cost to themselves emotionally – to conceal what was going on at the time? What right do we have to drag out from the records all these stories, whatever they may be, and broadcast them gleefully to our bemused or amused friends and relatives?

This is a question which, it could be said, particularly applies to those in the past who felt same-sex attraction. Nowadays, the vast majority of people would have nothing but sympathy for an ancestor who had a child out of wedlock, fell on hard times and ended up in the workhouse, shunned by her family. Not all researchers, however, might be as ready to tell the world about their great-great-uncle who ended up in prison because he was caught making love with his male partner, and his love letters were quoted in court as shaming evidence. There are two ways to deal with this. One is to accept that these people are long gone, that they were badly done by at the time, and now deserve to be posthumously 'out and proud' and we should feel proud of them too. Let us 'out' them, and celebrate their history!

The other way is to tell their stories, but as sensitively and honestly as possible and, where necessary, to do so with discretion. It is not this author's job to shock the reader with sensationalised accounts of individuals and their circumstances – to do so is not the approach of a responsible historian. In addition, to use tabloid tactics when telling this story is also to continue to sideline the subject of same-sex history to that of novelty or entertainment value and to continue to make the assumption that falling in love with the same gender is transgressive. It is not transgressive, but many people in history were treated as though it was. One would not shout to the world about a person's adoption if there is a possibility that they have not been told about it, as it could cause profound mental anguish. Similarly, I see no need to put the children or spouse of a recently deceased, covert homosexual in the same position. For this reason, I have a self-imposed privacy rule in place. All those, alive or recently deceased, who have so generously told their stories to the author and given permission for them to be included in this narrative, were given an undertaking that their names and other personal details would not be revealed. No attempt is made to hide away any stories, or fudge the issues involved. These are indeed stories that must, and should, be told, but it will be done with respect, affection and consideration.

CHAPTER ONE

Part I: Mollies, Catamites, Sapphists and Tribades – the Eighteenth Century

In 1700, England and Wales were about to leave behind a century that had been blighted by conflict, revolution, and religious, political and moral upheaval. The population was approximately five million, most of whom lived relatively isolated lives away from urban centres, such as they were then – London had a population of less than 450,000, approximately the size of Liverpool in the late twentieth century. It has been calculated that the news of King Charles I's execution in 1649 may have taken as long as two weeks to filter through to more remote parts of England and Wales, and half a century later the dissemination of intelligence, cultural changes and fashion was little better. Agricultural output was steady and the first signs of major industrial developments were manifesting themselves. In many communities, the Anglican parish church and its officers were still a major influence on the population, having an input into the administration of poor relief, registration of life events, revenue collection (tithes), and road repairs, not to mention attempts to keep the congregation on the moral straight and narrow path to Heaven.

In 1702, Queen Anne (1665–1714) ascended the throne. An ungainly woman with a dull husband, Anne had tragically suffered a long series of failed pregnancies, or very short lived live births, sixteen in all, plus one surviving child – William – who died in 1700 aged 11. With little in the way of political acumen she could not throw herself into her role as ruler either, and she was a lonely, grieving and somewhat derided figure. There was one thing in her life that did sustain her for many years, however – a passionate friendship with Sarah Churchill (nee Jennings, 1660–1744), later Duchess of Marlborough. Feisty, ambitious, attractive and intelligent, Sarah swept into Anne's life in the 1670s and brought lightness, loyalty, and affection, an emotional intimacy that the then princess craved; it was a closeness that lasted decades. They exchanged many letters, referring to each other

1

by pen names – Mrs Morley for the queen, and Mrs Freeman for Sarah. As a passionate champion of Anne's interests, Sarah was unpopular with some political factions, but she was unwavering in her support. One can never really know why another person's relationship starts to founder, but historians have deduced that Sarah's ambition for herself and her husband was the underlying reason why the two women parted company in about 1710 and Sarah and her husband were compelled to leave Court. Sarah had become dominating and blunt to the point of cruelty, her overriding ambition disillusioning the queen and her frequent voluntary absences from court distressing her. Anne turned to Sarah's cousin, Abigail Masham (nee Hill), as a replacement for the affection that had been snatched away from her. Abigail was gentle and kind to the ailing queen, a welcome change from the force of nature that was Sarah Churchill.

Was this friendship an *amor impossibilis*, or impossible love (a phrase used to describe a relationship between two women in early modern times)? It is not known if Anne and Sarah had any sexual element to their relationship, although the consensus leans towards it being passionate, but platonic. We deduce this from the letters the women exchanged, and from third party observations of what was going on. This relationship is a perfect example of the challenges of researching same-sex relationships, trying to tread the fine line between careless assumptions (or even wishful thinking) and presenting what facts we actually know or can deduce from archival sources, but the strictures of how we see same-sex relationships are also partly to blame for these limitations.

Another relationship, which occurred at about the same time, seemed to have fared better. In Westminster Abbey in London there is a beautiful monument to Mary Kendal, dated 1710. The lengthy inscription below the elegant sculpture of a praying Mary includes words celebrating 'the close Union and Friendship, In which she liv'd, with The Lady Catherine Jones; And in testimony of which she desir'd, That even their ashes, after Death, Might not be divided'.

Mrs MARY KENDALL daughter of Thomas Kendall Esqr. and of Mrs Mary Hallet, his wife, of Killigarth in Cornwall, was born at Westmr. [Westminster] Nov.8 1677 and dy'd at Epsome March 4 1709/10, having reach'd the full term of her blessed Saviour's life; and study'd to imitate his spotless example. She had great virtues, and as great a desire of concealing them: was of a severe life, but of an easy conversation; courteous to all, yet strictly sincere; humble, without meanness; beneficient, with-out ostentation; devout, without superstition. These admirable qualitys, in which she was equall'd by few of her sex, surpass'd by none, render'd her every way worthy of that close union and friendship in which she liv'd with the Lady CATHERINE JONES; and in testimony of which she desir'd that even their ashes, after death, might not be divided: and, therefore, order'd her selfe here to be interr'd where, she knew, that excellent Lady design'd one day to rest, near the grave of her belov'd and religious mother, ELIZABETH, Countess of RANELAGH. This monument was erected by Capt. CHARLES KENDALL.

How are we to define a same-sex relationship? If a survey were to be conducted today, there is no doubt that the majority of people would see a same-sex relationship as one based on a romantic or sexual attraction to a person of the same gender. That is the obvious answer because it seems to be human nature to assume a sexual element to all relationships, which are close or even passionate. However, if one accepts that the intimacy between Queen Anne and her friends is a same-sex relationship, then such a connection does not always have to be sexual to count. Human beings are capable of the greatest self-sacrifice, and can be vulnerable to love or intense feelings of affection for the same gender, whatever their sexuality.

Part II: Changing Attitudes Towards Male Same-sex Relationships

Leviticus 18:22 – Thou shalt not lie with mankind, as with womankind:
it [is] abomination.
(From the King James Bible)

It is sometimes suggested that the eighteenth century was a time of great change, scientifically, culturally, but also sexually, and that the contrast between the laissez-faire attitudes towards sex and relationships in the eighteenth century compared to the nineteenth century – particularly during the reign of Queen Victoria – is marked. Certainly, just as the Sapphic relationships between women were accepted to a degree, there were numerous different expressions of affection between men that were also, if not accepted, then at least tolerated. However, George Haggerty

3

wrote that there was a class difference in the way men were treated if they were discovered having a relationship with another man: 'A middle class gentleman may seduce a younger man and find himself in trouble (although only rarely and then he is usually acquitted), but a man of lower station may be executed for similar behaviour.' Certainly, as the eighteenth century progressed, it was no longer thought amusing or acceptable for a libertine or a rake, that is a man who was sexually promiscuous, to have intimacy with both males and females, so long as he was the dominant partner; many plays and comedies in the late seventeenth century clearly show that such sexual libertarianism was acceptable at that time. Whereas women of 'quality' were tolerated for having deep friendships with other women, even to the exclusion of other females, it was certainly not the case for men.

In 1700, 'the abominable vice of buggery' (anal intercourse) had been a criminal offence since 1533 and was also a capital offence, punishable by death. Yet many males had sexual contact with other males, from school age upwards, on a casual basis. Proximity of living, often sharing a bed, the lack of shaming labels, which were still over a century away, and the inherited, albeit diminishing, notion of the previous century that it was acceptable for a rake to have sex with either gender, all contributed to the culture of same-sex contact. Of course, Britons tried to attribute the origins of the 'vice' to foreigners; Turks, Russians and the Italians were blamed for its import into Britain, and it was labelled 'The Italian Vice', almost as if that nation had invented the practice (possibly a nod to the classical world and the mythical and other stories of men loving men that abound in classical literature, not to mention the influence of the Grand Tour, in which affluent young men travelled around places of cultural interest, taking in the remains of the classical world and sometimes bringing artefacts back home as 'souvenirs'). Not everyone tolerated this of course; in 1690, the Society for the Reformation of Manners was founded, with other moralistic groups following in the first third of the eighteenth century, which aimed to expose the haunts and activities of the sodomites (sodomy is another word for buggery) and 'mollies' (see below). Devout churchgoers and readers of the Bible – almost always the King James translation first published in 1611 but re-issued in 1769 with less elaborate English – would have noted the verses that seemed to condemn same-sex relationships (like that from Leviticus, above) and would have taken the view that male–male relationships in particular were not only illegal, but against God's wishes too.

4

CHAPTER ONE

Molly Houses

A molly house (from the Latin word mollia, meaning soft – as in foppish or effeminate) was a popular meeting place for men looking for social contact with other men, and in the eighteenth century there were plenty to choose from. The name was first used for the private club opened in 1709, the Mollies Club, which was established at a brandy house in Jermyn Street, London. Unfortunately the Mollies Club was shut down shortly afterwards and nine of the participators arrested and put on trial. However, its legacy was a continuing network of similar venues where men who desired men could meet and socialise. The 'mollies' themselves – largely those men who worked in the establishments but also some of those who frequented them – were seen as highly effeminate, with a liking for cross-dressing and a tendency to adopt the mannerisms of a particularly feminine woman, and it is likely that the majority of the mollies who resided in the premises were of working-class background. Their brazen appearances in public, sometimes at dances, dressed in elaborate women's clothing made them not only the target of assaults, but they were also likely to be arrested and charged as sodomists. One has to remember that these particular mollies are the ones we know about; their more masculine counterparts were less likely to be arrested and so went about their business and social lives more or less unhindered. Molly houses were essentially places for parties, romance and casual sexual encounters and their usual events bordered on the theatrical. It was not uncommon for mollies to go through a mock marriage ceremony with a client in the molly house before any sexual act took place – not necessarily to mimic a male–female relationship, where one was masculine and the other effeminate, but simply as a playful precursor to intimacy. If mollies were usually from a working-class or 'trade' background, their clientele could be from any walk of life. Middle- and upper-class men were more likely to have their masculinity undermined, it was suggested at the time, by too much tea-drinking, a 'soft' education, and a predilection for the opera! Consequently, there was a strange swapping of roles; mollies tended to put on airs and graces as if they were a great lady, and upper-class men were encouraged to avoid effeminacy and be more masculine and rugged, even if they desired other men. In 1726, a series of raids on certain establishments led to the discovery by the authorities of numerous molly houses, twenty being found in all. The most famous was that of Margaret 'Mother' Clap, based in Feld Lane, off Saffron Hill in Farringdon, London. Notoriety came with a price; twice, as punishment, she was put in shackles and taken to the pillories at Smithfield where she was locked into the contraption and pelted with dung, soil, stones, and all manner of rotting refuse helpfully supplied by the authorities. She also had to pay a hefty fine and was imprisoned for two years.

One man who, as a publican in London, seemed well placed to comment on the social scene there – however not as a client or a molly – was Edward 'Ned' Ward. Essentially a self-made man, he had some success with poetry writing and right at the end of the seventeenth century he started to produce a serial, *The London Spy*, which was finally published as a book in 1709. It was a witty, satirical, and sometimes damning, description of the colourful characters of London, some of whom must have been drinking customers of his – and one section of the part-work was about molly shops. One has to bear in mind that Ward is aiming to entertain and possibly even titillate his audience – this is not reportage – and so his account of what mollies did must be taken lightly, although his stories do seem to coincide with other contemporary accounts. Thus, Ward describes cross-dressing, and the assuming of a female persona:

> .... *imitating all the little Vanities that Custom has reconcil'd to the Female Sex, affecting to Speak, Walk, Tattle, Cursy* [i.e. curtsey], *Cry, Scold, and to mimick all Manner of Effeminacy, that ever has fallen within their several Observations; not omitting the Indecencies of Lewd Women, that they may tempt one another by such immodest Freedoms to commit those odious Bestialities, that ought for ever to be without a Name.*

The mollies, we are told, would take on the 'characters' of various women and gossip away in an exaggerated manner about the tribulations of their imagined lives with different types of husbands, such as the drunkard and the lazy man, whilst others complained about the tribulations of being single. Then:

> *No sooner had they ended their Feast, and run thro' all the Ceremonies of their Theatrical way of Gossiping, but, having wash'd away, with Wine, all fear of Shame, as well as the*

CHAPTER ONE

Checks of Modesty, then they began to enter upon their Beastly Obscenities, and to take those infamous Liberties with one another, that no Man, who is not sunk into a State of Devilism, can think on without Blushing, or mention without a Christian Abhorrence of all such Heathenish Brutalities.

Ward also repeats the stories about raucous re-enactments of the birth of a baby, with various mollies taking over-the-top parts of the labouring mother, the midwife, the church minister and so on, with a wooden doll taking the place of the newborn child. Clearly the mollies and their visitors have been included in the book as part of the weird and wonderful sights of the capital, but there is also plenty of fierce criticism there – just so the reader understands, perhaps, that Ward does not speak from personal experiences. It is really tabloid newspaper-reporting designed to sensationalise the private parties of a small minority of men who desired their own gender and, as he was a popular author, Ward would have influenced many to be as outraged as he apparently was. It is ironic that the 'recreation' of the birth of a baby, with all the exaggerated comedic play-acting involved, would have been highly amusing on the stage in a comedy at the time, but was deeply frowned upon as a private entertainment, especially as the mollies involved had no audience other than their own invited guests.

Although the molly houses made good copy and great entertainment, there were still plenty who wanted to see them eliminated. The Societies for the Reformation of Manners were the initiators of many of the raids on the molly shops, and any subsequent prosecutions were filled with shocked descriptions of what went on in the establishments. At the trial of Gabriel Lawrence, a 43-year-old milkman indicted for committing sodomy with 30-year-old wool-comber Thomas Newton at Mother Clap's molly house, informing agent Samuel Stevens described what he had seen:

I have been several times, in order to detect those who frequented it: I have seen 20 or 30 of them together, kissing and hugging, and making Love (as they call it) in a very indecent Manner. Then they used to go out by Couples into another Room, and, when they came back, they would tell what they had been doing, which, in their Dialect, they called Marrying.

Both the above men were working class and as such, vulnerable to the worst that the law could throw at them; as George Haggerty suggested, had many of those apprehended at molly houses been of better social rank, they would have escaped the worst of the punishment. Like many other people who had same-sex desires over the centuries, the men who frequented molly shops were often married – Gabriel Lawrence was married twice, and both his fathers-in-law testified on his behalf at his trial. One has to look at the times to put this and many other marriages into perspective. To have a spouse was almost like having an essential helper, companion and, as it was put at that time, 'helpmeet' – an economic and pragmatic necessity and a fulfilment of what God demanded – to marry and procreate. Any children from a marriage were an essential economic unit, often needed to keep the family afloat, providing both wages and labour from an early age. Marriage was the height of respectability and perhaps the men who went through these mock marriages at the molly houses were subconsciously expressing a need, or desire, to make their same-sex relationships just as respectable; or perhaps they were mocking a society that would not allow them to join its 'respectable' ranks if openly living with a same-sex partner and trying to make their way in life as a couple. Of course, one must be careful not to see these eighteenth century activities in the light of twenty-first century marriage equality, a concept which a man at that time may well have found anathema, even if he was a sodomite himself. One can see, however, a widespread public horror of any lampooning of the married state, acceptable if it is about a man and a woman and conducted by a 'respectable' cartoonist or playwright – but totally unacceptable if by sodomites in a molly house. This distinction helped drive many more men into covert liaisons, afraid as they were not only of the law, but of public scorn and disgust; it is also a portent of the Victorian mania for respectability that was to come in the following century.

The targeting of molly houses must have been a deterrent for many men who feared being apprehended there, and men often continued to find their pleasures in other ways. Chance encounters, taverns that turned a blind-eye to a man making the acquaintance of another man, and even, ostensibly, heterosexual brothels that hosted same-sex liaisons also existed. Some may have met their lovers in the course of their work or just through casual social acquaintance – in October 1722, the *Stamford Mercury* reported on the trial for sodomy of Thomas Pococke of Oxford, a fruiterer:

it appeared he was aged 72 Years, and had practised that abom-
inable Vice near 20 Years, which was proved by 5 Witnesses; the
most notorious was in June last, with the Tapster at the Angel.
The Fact was clearly proved, and the Jury found him Guilty.

In November 1730, two men in London found an altogether different
venue for their casual encounter – St Paul's Cathedral. At the trial of
William Holiwell and William Huggins, a waterman, the witness John
Rowden (who seems to be a guide at the cathedral) stated that as he was
going to his lunch break he came across the two prisoners in a highly
compromising position. Whilst Huggins desperately tried to pull his
clothes back on, Rowden quickly locked the door to the side aisle, the main
way out of that area, but Holiwell still tried to get away, struggling with
Rowden and tearing his clothes. Holiwell did escape but was apprehended
in another part of the cathedral and the two men were arrested. Apart
from the crucial witness who claimed he had seen the two men in the
process of a sexual act, 'tokens of emissions' on the shirt of Holiwell
were taken as further proof that intimacy had taken place. Holiwell did
not bring forward any character witnesses for himself, but his lover,
Huggins, produced several, who all praised the devoted family man for
being a very hard worker, honest in business, and a regular churchgoer –
in fact, they all claimed, he was the last person they expected to be in
such a predicament. It was also pointed out how at ease he was in female
company and that he preferred that to the friendship of men. Having been
found guilty of misdemeanour – Holiwell for assaulting his lover with
intent to commit sodomy, and Huggins for submitting to the 'assault' –
they both suffered spells in the pillory, Holiwell spent six months in
prison and paid a £40 fine (approximately £3,400 in modern terms), and
Huggins spent eight months in prison. Perhaps the latter was spared a
fine because he was the 'receiver' in the encounter and also because such
a financial blow could destroy his family, the innocent victims of the
court case.

There was therefore widespread disapproval of the 'Italian vice',
and there was sufficient public interest in it for the street-ballad writers
to pen verses about it. In 1707, The Women-Hater's Lamentation was
published, following several raids on molly houses, and the subsequent
suicides of some of the men awaiting trial. Some of the fourteen verses
go as follows:

SAME SEX LOVE 1700–1957

I
Ye injured females see
Justice without the laws, Seeing the injury,
Has thus reveng'd your cause.

IV
Nature they lay aside,
To gratify their lust;
Women they hate beside,
Therefore their fate was just.

VII
But see the fateful end
That do's such Crimes pursue;
Unnat'al Deaths attend,
Unnat'ral lusts in you.

X
A Hundred more we hear,
Did to this club belong;
But now they scatter'd are,
For this has broke the gang.

XI
Shopkeepers some there were,
And some of good repute,
Each vow'd a batchelor,
Unnat'ral Lust purs'd.

XIV
This piece of justice then
Has well reveng'd their Cause,
And shews unnat'ral Lust
Is cursed without the laws.

CHAPTER ONE

As the eighteenth century progressed, executions of men accused of sodomy continued. In the second half of the 1700s, approximately one man per decade was executed in London, and one each year in Middlesex. Ironically, in many cases it was difficult to prove sodomy had taken place, so it was easier for the authorities to secure a conviction on the grounds of assault with the intent to commit sodomy (the basis of the Holiwell/ Huggins trial, above). Penalties for this misdemeanour were between one month and two years in gaol, or being placed in the pillory. Sometimes the mob took matters into its own hands, actually killing a man they suspected of sodomy in 1780. Others were shocked by this mob rule and Edmund Burke proposed the abolition of the pillory to the House of Commons, although unfortunately this was not to happen until the nineteenth century.

Anti-same-sex literature also started to appear. Works with sensationalist titles like *Satan's Harvest Home: or the Present State of Whorecraft, Adultery, Fornication, Procuring, Pimping, Sodomy, And the Game of Flatts, (Illustrated by an Authentick and Entertaining Story) And other Satanic Works, daily propagated in this good Protestant Kingdom* (1749) warned of the growing peril of the vice both in men and women. Boys, we are told, were being raised by fussy mothers with masculine influences elbowed aside, so that the next generation of men were growing up effeminate weaklings:

> ... *his Mamma had charged him not to play with rude Boys, for fear of spoiling his Cloathes; so that hitherto our young gentleman has amused himself with Dolls, assisted at mock Christenings, and other girlish employments, inviting and being invited to drink Tea with this or that School-fellow.*
>
> [when the 'mother's boy' grows up] *What satisfaction can a Woman have in the embraces of this Figure of a Man?* [the resulting child would be a] *feeble, unhealthy infant, scarce worth the rearing; whilst the Father, instead of being the head of the Family, makes it seem as if it were governed by two Women ...... Unfit to serve his King, his Country, or his Family, this Man of Clouts dwindles into nothing, and leaves his race as effeminate as himself; who, unable to please the Women, chuse rather to run into unnatural Vices one with another.*

How could such fops, asks the author, be capable of dominating women when they themselves had grown up dominated by females? There is a sly reference here to the molly house, perhaps, in the reference to mock christenings, which would not have been lost on the readership of the day. In short, the author is warning of the growth of a generation of soft-fleshed, cowardly, feminised males. This is not the only hint of what was to come either – this work smacks of eugenics, the careful guarding of the family unit against unhealthy influences and the moulding of future generations by selective breeding. Here there is also the idea that a relationship with a man is chosen because the effeminate male cannot satisfy his wife – in other words, he is inferior in a number of ways.

Whilst this all sounds far fetched now, there were plenty of middle-class, God-fearing families who would have taken this pamphlet very seriously, and it is an interesting foreshadowing of the theories of the sexologists in the nineteenth and twentieth centuries.

Little wonder then, that William Beckford, the richest man in England, fled the country and remained in self-imposed exile in Europe for ten years when rumours started circulating in 1784 about his liaison with a younger male, William 'Kitty' Courtenay, 9th Earl of Devon, in what became known as the 'Powderham Affair' (after Kitty's property, Powderham Castle). Kitty was an extremely beautiful young man known for his same-sex desires, and the two men were caught in a compromising situation by Kitty's uncle, Lord Loughborough. Loughborough was so incensed that he went out of his way to ruin Beckford, who was only 25 years old at the time; he was to live another sixty years with the stigma of this scandal.

Part III: Passions Between Women

Meanwhile, there is ample evidence of women falling in love with each other or having passionate encounters – or simply just deeply bonded friendships. William King (1685–1763) wrote *The Toast* in 1736, which referred to the Duchess of Newburgh as a lesbian. Exactly what he meant by this is unclear, but as one of the few words in use today that has survived the centuries to describe people with same-sex feelings, it certainly implies romantic or women-oriented relationships. Other terms used to describe women who were attracted to women were 'tribade' (from tribadism, a word from the Greek used to describe a sexual act) and 'frictrice' (from the Latin word *frico*, meaning to rub or chafe), and the act of making love was also known as 'the flats'. *Satan's Harvest Home* tells us that the fault lies squarely with Sappho and her poetry, and that the 'the flats', or tribadism, was originally from Turkey and also caused by public bathing. Romantic, even passionate, friendships were common amongst women who could not otherwise express their feelings for other women, and the story of Elizabeth Carter is a typical one. Born in 1717 in Kent, the daughter of a vicar, she was well educated at home in languages and music, and at the age of 21 she began to publish small pieces, firstly in the *Gentleman's Magazine*, under the pen name 'Eliza'; these were followed by a booklet of poems, *Poems on Particular Occasions*. It is no surprise, therefore, that the romantic feelings Elizabeth had for her closest friend, Catherine Talbot, were expressed through her writing, in this case in letters to Catherine. They found each other in 1741, but had little personal time together – Catherine was an invalid, cared for by her mother. A translation of the works of the Greek philosopher Epictetus was so well received that Elizabeth was able to live independently on the proceeds, and devote her time to nurturing her thirty-year romance with Catherine.

After Catherine died in 1770, Elizabeth made the acquaintance of the Bluestockings, female intellectuals such as Elizabeth Montagu, and she also knew other great thinkers of the day such as Fanny Burney. Catherine's mother left a bequest to Elizabeth that enabled her to continue to live independently till her death in 1806, a gesture that suggests she valued the feelings Elizabeth had for her daughter and did not think ill of them.

A contemporary of Elizabeth Carter's was not quite so pure in her love for other women, however. Charlotte Charke (1713–1760) was the daughter of none other than the Poet Laureate, Colley Cibber, and grew up a boisterous and very active child who swaggered round the house in her brother's clothes and her father's wig. She married twice, as was expected of her, but her first husband deserted her and the second marriage was also short lived. As an independent woman she had a colourful life with numerous jobs, which included a pastry, cook, grocer, oil-selling business and puppet show, and she also took masculine parts in various London shows, acting as Hamlet, Mercury and Captain Plume, as well as MacHeath in the *Threepenny Opera* at the Haymarket in 1744. She had an equally assertive approach to her female conquests, but the woman she set up home with is respectfully referred to in Charlotte's memoirs (published 1755) as 'Mrs Brown'. When the couple went to live in Bristol, Charlotte passed as male (wore male attire and 'performed' the role of a man in public), which she described as being 'en cavalier', and the locals accepted the couple as man and wife; it was as an established couple that 'Mr and Mrs Brown' returned to live in London after yet another failed business venture. Charlotte died in poverty in 1760, it is thought with her beloved 'Mrs' by her side; at least in her final years she had the domestic love she had seemingly been looking for in her youth.

Other women in the eighteenth century also made no secret of their love for another female, but even if one was affluent and well connected it did not guarantee success in courtship. The renowned sculptor Anne Damer (1749–1828) was passionately in love with Mary Berry (1763–1852), who lived with her sister in Twickenham. Mary never allowed Anne's advances to stray beyond the preliminaries and kept her suitor at arm's length, as a friend only. Anne turned her attentions to actress Elizabeth Farren, the future Countess of Derby, and their affair was lampooned in satirical street pamphlets, with ribald speculation that Anne did a lot more for Elizabeth sexually than her husband ever could.

The attempts to categorise people with different sexualities at this time were born out of a struggle to understand. If tribades and sodomites are ostensibly women and men – how could they be? They did not feel and act like 'normal' God-fearing people – then what were they? Some said they were hermaphrodites, a special type of person somewhere in between the two genders and with unclear, or two types of, genitalia – what may now be referred to as intersexed, but it is impossible that all the women who had same-sex relationships were intersexed, simply on the grounds of probability.

Female Husbands, Passing Women and Sapphic Marriages

I

If you want to hear a bit of fun,
Oh listen unto me,
About a Female Husband,
The like you never see,
Such a singular thing you never knew,
No not in all your life,
As two females to be wed,
And live as Man and Wife.
Chorus

CHAPTER ONE

So young women all a warning take,
And mark what I do say,
Before you wed, your husbands try,
Or else you'll rue the day.

II
The Female Husband lived
In service as a Groom'Twas there that she got wed,
To the housemaid in her bloom,
At Camberwell the truth I tell,
The Wedding was, it's true,
You'll laugh till all is blue.

III
The parties they were shown to bed,
The bride sir, thought of that,
But the bridegroom he was taken ill,
Made everything look flat,
From his bride he turn'd and twisted.
Then she to herself did say,
My husband is a Hermaphrodite,
A wager I would lay.

VII
Sometime he was a sawyer,
Done his duty like a man,
'Twas there his days were ended,
As you shall understand.
There was not one as we could hear,
Did of his manhood doubt,
But now it's o'er he is no more,
And the secret is found out.

VIII
Now for Twenty years they lived,
As man and wife so clever,
Both eat and drank, and slept,
And just these things together;

15

If women all could do the same,
And keep their virgin know,
Why the King and all his subjects,
Would quickly go to pot.

X

So I do advise young women all,
To look before you wed,
For if you should be so deceived,
You will rue your marriage bed.

(Extracts from the street ballad of 1828–9, *The Female Husband*)

Anyone who tried to 'pass' as another gender was going to be vulnerable to exposure, either in their lifetime – due to illness or a brush with the law – or after their death. Many women who dressed in male clothes did so because of the practicalities of doing dirty or strenuous work, or were following beloved husbands or fathers into a war or similarly masculine environment and that necessitated passing as male to be in close proximity to loved ones. Other women did so purely from a sense of adventure, not wishing to be restricted by the social and cultural constraints of their gender; yet more, whether interested in same-sex relationships or not, passed as male for fraudulent purposes, and targeted – sometimes wooed – women known to have savings in order to have access to the money. As well as the above cross-dressing women such as Charlotte Charke, there are plentiful examples of other women who dressed as men, took a man's job and also had relationships or even marriages with other women. It is unclear exactly how many there were, because the ones historians discover are those who hit the headlines or ended up in the courtroom for some reason. Such women were known as female husbands in their lifetime, and are now also sometimes referred to as passing women – literally passing as male as a sort of disguise, safety measure or expression of something in their sexuality or gender that in their day would have had no name and no explanation.

Mary 'George' Hamilton was one of these women. Born in approximately 1721, she came to light having been arrested under the Vagrancy Act in 1776, 'for having by false and deceitful practices endeavoured to impose on some of his Majesty's subjects.' It was claimed that whilst posing as a physician she had tricked two women at least about her gender when starting relationships with them, and indeed, married two of them; in court it was also alleged that a dildo was found in her belongings and this was shown as evidence of her intent to deceive. 'George' was found guilty, publicly whipped in four market towns and imprisoned for six months. Author Henry Fielding was so intrigued by this case that he wrote a partly fictionalised account of it in his pamphlet *The Female Husband*, published in 1746. Readers fascinated by this tale could then enjoy the story of Italian sapphist Catherine Vizzani, an English edition of which was published in 1751. She had begun her romantic relationships with women in her teens, and before long was passing as male to the point where she ended up being shot in a dispute with a man over a woman. The author concluded that Catherine had somehow been perverted by listening to inappropriate stories.

Ann Marrow was convicted of fraud in the following year for 'going in men's clothes, and personating a man in marriage with three different women ... defrauding them of their money and effects.' She was sentenced to three months in gaol and had to stand in the pillory at Charing Cross, where she was blinded in both eyes because of the severity with which she was pelted with stones. Another famous example, which elicited a more sympathetic response from the public both locally and further afield, was that of James How, aka Mary East. In 1766 she and her 'wife' were revealed in the *Gentleman's Magazine* as having lived together for over thirty years as spouses in Poplar, with Mary adopting the husband's role in both employment and attire. They had done well for themselves, running a successful inn, the White Horse, and saving up £3,000 from their hard work and enjoying 'good credit and esteem'. Unfortunately, an old acquaintance recognised Mary despite the cross-dressing and over the course of fifteen years, tried twice to blackmail her, in 1765 sending men to beat Mary as she had refused to pay. James (Mary) confided the situation to a male friend and the blackmailer and one of the attackers were brought to court and sent to gaol. It is pleasing to read that the local community rallied round the two female spouses, appearing in court as character witnesses. Two points are worthy of note here. Firstly, the magazine is at pains to point out that the two women only entered into their relationship because they had been let down as young women by male partners; and secondly, that they were regarded as having a good name with their neighbours even after the story was exposed. Such statements would ensure that any accusations of sapphism – a sexual element to the bond the two women must surely have had – would be deflected as suggestions of abnormality might undermine the sympathies of the reader.

How many women cross-dressed, or passed as men, in order to live with their female partner unhindered? We will never know. It is also clear that many women did not feel the need, for whatever reason, to conceal their relationship, and in the rural North East Cheshire parish of Taxal, two extraordinary entries in the parish register, if correct, are testament to this. It is unlikely that in the next example, any of the four women in question tried to pass as male; they certainly kept their female names in any case. On 4 September 1707, Hannah Wright and Anne Gaskill were married – to each other, and the parish register clearly records the event along with all the other life events it dealt with. The following year, 1708, Ane (probably Ann/e) Norton and Alice Pickford were married at the same church on 3 June, and again the parish register clearly records the event apart from an unusual spelling of the first name Ane.

A closer look at the parish register reveals more details. On 25 February 1706, an Alice Pickford married one Jona (probably Jonathan) Swan. If this is the Alice who later married a woman, why did she marry again in 1708 using her birth surname and not her married name, which, if she was a widow by then, she would normally have kept? An Alice Pickford died in May 1731 and was buried on the twenty-eighth of that month, but does not appear to have left a will, which as a widow or single woman, she could have done (bearing in mind her marriage to a woman, if it occurred, would not have been legally recognised). Again, if this burial is 'our' Alice, why was she not using the name of her spouse, An(n)e Norton – An(n)e's name was first in the parish register, so that implies she was taking the role of the groom. The Alice who married Jonathan Swan was from Prestbury, another Cheshire village approximately nine miles away. In both places, there is evidence of Pickford families and it is likely that the two family groups are related at some level. Then again, another Alice Pickford died in Prestbury and was buried on 20 June 1722. Will the Alice who married An(n)e Norton please step forward?

Gaskill, in various spellings of that name, is a common Cheshire and Derbyshire surname, and there are certainly numerous Gaskills in Taxal at around the time of the two marriages. There is also evidence of Nortons and Wrights in Taxal in previous years, but not to the same extent as the other names. Swan does not seem to be a name common to these villages.

CHAPTER ONE

Unfortunately, none of these ponderings lead us to any information at present that would throw light on these four women. So what can we conclude about these events? We could take them at face value and accept that here we have two Sapphic marriages which the minister or curate for some reason has allowed to take place. It has been suggested by other researchers that these women may have travelled to the parish especially to marry, but this is unlikely, bearing in mind the presence of the surnames in the parish registers over many years, as proven by a survey of the registers from their beginnings in 1610 to the end of the eighteenth century. It is reasonable, therefore, to surmise that the women are known locally, possibly even born in the village or close by, and that one at least may have been conventionally married. It may be that these 'marriages' were a unique local way of acknowledging that these women were going to live together as an economic unit and were thus unavailable for marriage or remarriage to a man. The fact that the events are so far back in the records creates its own issues, as every family historian will acknowledge. All four women were more than likely illiterate, and there is no evidence of their having any property – certainly none of them left wills, although only Alice's burial can be identified and we don't know when and where the other three died. In an area where so many had the same surnames and first names, building a solid life story for any one of them is a complex undertaking, and we are pretty much left with the marriage entries themselves, especially as the Bishop's Transcripts are missing for those years and we do not have their corroboration – but if the marriages were as they appear at face value, would they have been copied into the Bishop's Transcript for Diocesan superiors to see? Were the entries a joke or a sly form of bullying or intimidation, written in the register without the knowledge of the minister, because the women were known to have a bond? The honest answer is we do not know; all we can say for sure is that there were people with same-sex desires everywhere, in all levels of society, and that part of Cheshire would have been no different. What changes from era to era, and place to place, and social group to social group, is how that desire manifests itself, not whether it exists or not.

Sadly, women who tried to marry covertly did not always have the same good fortune as our ladies in Taxal, despite their efforts to be discreet. In the parish register for Bolton Percy, near York, a marriage entry from January 1756/7, which on the surface seems perfectly in order, has been very determinedly crossed out, the strong criss-cross of lines on the page making it clear that this entry was to be ignored. The marriage was between John Brown, a labourer, and Anne Steel, who was from a large local family. Banns had been read and no objection to the marriage had been made at the time, so it went ahead as arranged. There is no note explaining why this 'cancellation' had been done, and were it not for a copy of the register presented to the Archbishop – the Bishop's Transcript –, we would still not know the complete story. Thankfully, the copy of the entry has also been carefully crossed out in the transcript, and the following explanation given: 'afterwards discovered to be a woman dressed in man's apparel and of course separated from the said Ann Steel.'

It is now thought that 'John Brown' was in fact the same person who was discovered in York to be Barbara Hill, a local woman who had left York after working as a servant there, and who returned to enlist in the army. Unfortunately, someone recognised her despite her male presentation and revealed her gender to the officers, who of course immediately discharged her. The newspapers delighted in telling their readers that John Brown's 'supposed wife' also arrived in York, begging that they stay together. By way of explanation, Barbara said that when she had left York the first time, she had also left her female clothes behind and, travelling south, became apprenticed to a stonecutter. She also worked as a farmer and a coach-driver before making her way back home to the North again.

It is unlikely that there would be two passing women by the name of John Brown in such a close proximity to each other, so it is reasonable to assume that Ann Steel's lover was Barbara Hill. Possibly someone recognised Barbara yet again, and exposed the fraud (the whole thing could have ended up in both the church and secular courts), but whatever the course of events, we do know that Ann married again in 1765, ironically to another Browne, this time a William. This is about nine years after her first marriage to John/Barbara. Were the two women able to get together again in these intervening years, facing down the local gossips and scandal, or did Ann have to wait until the local tittle-tattle had stopped before seeking security with a man? We do not know, and we cannot say what happened to Barbara either, as she disappears from the records after 1760. It would be comforting to think that despite the comment in the register, their relationship did not collapse under the weight of all that disapproval, and that it lasted at least some time after they were exposed.

CHAPTER ONE

Female husbands, or passing women, whatever description is used, are basically this: women who dressed as men. It is known that many women, frustrated by the restrictions of society, assumed a male identity to pursue better-paid work in order to maintain a household. Of these, a sizeable number – more than likely the majority – had female partners, whom they sometimes married in a church without the clergyman realising anything untoward. The reason that female husbands feature so strongly in narratives such as this, is that it is one of the few ways we can access stories about female same-sex relationships – they hit the headlines at the time, just as men did because they broke the law, and so we have many such tales to look at. Female husbands and their wives tend also to be working class, and this is again an area that we would find it hard to describe without these tales.

In 1748 and 1749, John Cleland published *Memoirs of a Woman of Pleasure*, more popularly known as *Fanny Hill*. The reminiscences of a reformed prostitute told in the first person, the story caused a sensation in its day, and the Bishop of London, Thomas Sherlock, pressurised the Secretary of State to issue a warrant for Cleland's arrest; the subsequent prosecution led to a prison sentence for Cleland and a £100 fine. Although the story is significant for its insights into eighteenth century sexuality as a whole, it is also important for the insights it offers into some popular views about same-sex relationships. In the story, Fanny witnesses two men making love and whereas the rest of the novel titillates the reader with, rather than condemns sexual freedoms, in this instance we are left in no doubt that Fanny is appalled by what she sees – as she says 'so criminal a scene' is disgusting to her. In fact, although this is said for dramatic effect, Fanny is right – as the two men were engaging in anal intercourse, they were indeed committing an illegal act and they faced the harshest punishments. Also, in a comment reminiscent of the mania for looking for identifying marks on witches one hundred years previously, Fanny's employer, Mrs Cole, insists that the English climate was conducive to such practices but that these men would be left with a distinguishing mark – a 'plague spot' – which would presumably be very convenient for those trying to identify or reject those who were not suitable marriage candidates. Looking at the situation from the point of view of a woman at the time, the majority of females sought out a husband who would bring them the security they needed to survive with the brood of children they would more than likely produce, and a man whose focus was not entirely on supporting his family unit was an economic and social threat.

However, it is very difficult to assess exactly what Cleland's true agenda was in writing this novel and including same-sex themes in it. Was he trying to make fun of people with such condemnatory opinions by articulating them through the amoral Fanny, who, as she looks back on her past exploits, is more prudish than some religious fanatics? Cleland could just as easily be making fun of the moral high ground, as siding with it, but he must have taken his ideas from opinions and events he encountered in his everyday life.

Hot on the heels of Fanny Hill (in a manner of speaking) was the pamphlet *Ancient and Modern Pederasty Investigated and Exemplify'd*, written by one Thomas Cannon. Cannon and Cleland were known to each other (in fact Cleland owed Cannon £800) and Cleland denounced Cannon as a 'molly' in an offensive note left at the latter's place of work; Cannon claimed to be a scholar of the history of male–male relationships going right back to ancient times, and from the excerpts that have survived it would seem that the author's aim was to place these relationships at the heart of history, in a sense, normalising them. Unfortunately, as a prosecution was imminent, Cannon and his publisher had to flee the country, but this drastic action was not typical of writers of such tracts at the time, and they were by no means illicit texts.

There has never been a time when all those who fell in love with someone of their own gender could shirk their other responsibilities, whether marital or otherwise. Lord John Hervey (1696–1743), a slightly built man who presented as very effeminate, to the point where he was lampooned by famous writers such as Alexander Pope, was the eldest son of the 1st Earl of Bristol, and had a conventional life in many ways. He graduated from Cambridge, did the Grand Tour as all young men of his status did, married (and fathered eight children), and became a Member of Parliament – altogether the standard life of a privileged man of his day. It was presumably through parliamentary circles that he met his great love, Stephen Fox (1704–1776), a fellow MP. Duties at the royal court often kept the two men apart, much to Hervey's dismay and regret; 'I can't live without you', he wrote to Fox. The affair was known to Hervey's wife, who in fact liked her 'rival' and looked to him for news of her husband. There was little point her objecting in any case; she would have been brought up to accept that men of Hervey's status had what amounted to a patriarchal right to extra-marital relationships, and at least the third person in the triangle was not going to present her with the problem of an illegitimate child!

Interestingly, despite being well known about, the affair did not prevent Hervey's career in public life from flourishing. In 1733 Hervey took the title Baron Hervey and entered the House of Lords, became Lord Privy Seal in 1740 and advanced Fox's career too at the same time as helping Fox with his marriage plans – a marriage that also saw the end of their long standing affair. In 1736, he also had an affair with Count Francesco Algarotti, who may well have been his last lover before his death in 1743.

The Ladies of Llangollen

> In ours, the Vale of Friendship, let *this* spot
> Be named; where, faithful to a low-roofed Cot,
> On Deva's banks, ye have abode so long;
> Sisters in love, a love allowed to climb,
> Even on this earth, above the reach of time!

(William Wordsworth; extract from his 1824 sonnet *To the Lady E.B. and the Hon. Miss P.,* written in honour of the Ladies of Llangollen and to celebrate their love for each other)

In 1778, two women arrived in Llangollen, North Wales, and took over the run down Plas Newydd, a charming black and white property in what was then a fairly out of the way part of the country, certainly at a distance from the prying eyes and chattering gossips of the main upper- and middle-class venues such as Bath and London. Eleanor Butler (1739–1829) and Sarah Ponsonby (1755–1831) had fallen deeply in love ten years before, and escaped the disapproval of their families in Ireland, travelling to Llangollen to set up home together.

There has always been an opinion that the two women were much more than simply romantic friends, but other historians have argued that such a relationship could not have been sexual; this may be a legacy of their family's refusal to accept that they could be doing no more than holding hands and reading poetry to each other! The fact is, we do not know. They addressed each other as 'my better half' and 'my beloved', shared a bed and their income, signed letters jointly, received visitors as a couple (including Anne Lister, [see below] who saw them as a couple in a marriage such as she would have with a woman), named one of their dogs Sappho, and in every way, lived as life-partners. It may have been in their interests to play down any physical side to their relationship in order to have a better social life and more contact with a wider circle, but it really does not matter if they physically made love to each other or not. What cannot be denied is that they lived devotedly with each other for fifty years, only parted by death when Eleanor passed away first, in 1829, at the age of ninety. Sarah survived her for about twelve months. They are buried side by side in the local church graveyard.

CHAPTER TWO

The Nineteenth Century

Whereas the Ladies of Llangollen managed to stay largely on the right side of public approval, two school teachers in Scotland ended up the wrong side of the law thanks to an accusation by one of their young pupils. The scandal hit the headlines all over Britain and must have made other women in the same position of responsibility think very carefully about how they conducted themselves. In 1810, Jane Pirie and Marianne Woods were accused by Jane Cumming, one of their pupils, of engaging in intimate acts together, which the girl claimed to have heard. The women apparently lay on top of each other, kissed and fondled, and the bed shook. On one occasion, Pirie was reported to have whispered to Woods, 'Oh, do it darling'. The child also said she heard a noise like 'putting one's finger into the neck of a wet bottle'. To what must have been the overwhelming relief of the two women, the judges were largely unimpressed. One said: 'Are we to say that every woman who has formed an intimate friendship and has slept in the same bed as another is guilty? Where is the innocent woman in Scotland?' What then had to be decided was if the women had gone from friendship to something considered more inappropriate. Clearly the idea of close – even physically intimate – bonds between women was, if not encouraged, then certainly accepted at this time, which may be why the Ladies of Langollen chose to present their relationship in the way they did. This was after all the age of the Romantics.

The nineteenth century began for sodomites as it had been continuing before, with executions of men who had been convicted of sodomy. In 1804, Mathusala Spalding was hanged for the crime, another five men were hanged in Lancaster and in 1808, a Joshua Archer was also hanged. In 1808, the Home Secretary, Lord Liverpool, ordered Hyde Park and St James's Park in London to be closed at night, in order to protect the public from the nocturnal activities in them.

The Vere Street Scandal

The White Swan on Vere Street in London – essentially a molly house – was a very popular if disorderly venue for largely working-class men, from all different walks of life, and had been established by James Cook and a man by the name of Yardley. Unlike some other molly houses, this seemed to have many working-class, often married, men as clientele, and a variety of facilities were available for the 'guests' to enjoy themselves together. Some men would cross-dress on specific occasions, and examples given at the time were the likes of an 'athletic bargeman', who when cross-dressing was known as Fanny Murry; and a well-built coal heaver who adopted the name Lucy Cooper. However, this relatively safe environment was soon to be exposed. In July 1810, having only been open for about six months, the establishment was raided and twenty-three men were taken away – eight men were convicted and sentenced to between one and three years in gaol. The convicted men were transported through a dangerous and jeering crowd and then placed in the pillory to be pelted by the usual filth, manure and even dead animals, which could cut and maim their faces and damage eyesight. The aim was not to effect a 'cure' of the men's desires, but to punish the act and deter them and others from doing it again; literally, making a public example of them. James Cook was subjected to a particularly vicious level of aggression because of his strong, masculine appearance and his refusal to break under the pressure of the assault and behave like a molly (that is in an effeminate manner by crying and trying to hide away) and when at the end, he still refused to cower in the filth on the floor, he was whipped by a coachman. Clearly it was not his penitence people wanted to see, but the abjection of a warped personality, duly chastened. Thomas White, aged 16, and John Hepburn, aged 44, were convicted of buggery and hanged, despite apparently not being on the premises at the time of the raid. No doubt the other men breathed a sigh of relief that there was insufficient evidence against them – although the damage to their work, businesses and family life must have been punishment enough.

However, no matter what was done as deterrent, men and women were going to make close bonds with their own gender. In 1815, a scandal aboard HMS *Africaine* led to four sailors being hanged for sodomy; stories in the provincial newspapers appeared regularly detailing sodomites who had been apprehended. In Warrington in 1806, the *Chester Courant* of

6 May reported that 'a numerous gang of sodomites' were arrested and four were sent for trial at Lancaster Assizes; they included three men from Warrington itself, John Knight, a glass maker; Isaac Hitchen, a 62-year-old baker; Joshua Newsome, a 34-year-old servant; and Samuel Stockton, a 50-year-old whitster (cloth-bleacher) from nearby Latchford. The men had clearly formed some kind of social club, it was said, based upon a Masonic lodge, and the members called each other 'Brother'. Some of the men were affluent, such as 50-year-old Joseph Holland, and it was presumably the wealthier men in the group who secured the property kept expressly for their meetings, with Hitchin as caretaker. Holland was accused of committing 'an unnatural crime' upon Warrington man, Thomas Taylor, as was Samuel Stockton. Other men in the group included Thomas Rix, aged 47; Peter Atherton, aged 72; and John Hebden Constantine.

Between 1800 and 1834, eighty men were hanged in England for sodomy. A clerical victim of scandal, the Bishop of Clogher from Northern Ireland fled when released on bail in 1822 after being found literally with his breeches round his ankles with John Moverley, a Grenadier guardsman, in a public house in Haymarket, London. It is thought that he ended up in Scotland, and died in obscurity; he was of course removed from his office and replaced. It was important for men to protect their good names from any imputation of same-sex activity; it was not just a matter of good name, but may even have meant facing a life or death trial if it went that far. In Kent in 1813, John Silver sought damages against Francis Cobb, a brandy merchant, for defamation. Silver was an eminent surgeon and according to his counsel had the 'most irreproachable character'; he was married and had fathered nine children. Silver had applied to join a music club in Margate, but a number of existing members had voted against his application and it was rejected. Having seen the vote, Cobb declared that if they did have Silver as a member 'They might as well elect Tommy Hughes'. Tommy Hughes, says the newspaper, was a local man who was 'addicted to sodomitical practices' (*Kent Weekly Post or Canterbury Journal*, 23 March) although he does not seem to have been prosecuted for sodomy. When the comments were made known to Silver, he immediately took action to protect his good name from this 'scandalous aspersion'. Despite the insistence of the defendant that he had not meant such a slur, the jury found in Silver's favour and Cobb was fined £50. In 1828 it was made easier for a prosecution to prove that a sexual act had taken place between two men by lessening the evidence required. In 1833, Captain Henry Nichols was hanged at Horsemonger Lane Gaol in Southwark, for his 'heinous, horribly frightful, and disgusting crime' of desiring another man. He died knowing that his family had abandoned him completely, refusing to visit him in gaol; they also refused to claim his body after the execution. William John Bankes had to resign from parliament in 1834 after he was arrested by police for having a relationship with a soldier in the Royal Guards. In 1836, the Criminal Law Committee considered whether or not to remove sodomy from the list of capital crimes and decided it was too vile to be removed. Consequently, another 200 men were hanged between 1836 and 1856 for committing the crime of 'giving in' to their desires in an increasingly moralistic society. Middle- and working-class families must have shaken their heads over their newspapers and family bibles, and worried for their own family members who didn't seem interested in getting married, or whose involvement with certain 'friends' could eventually cause them to end up in gaol, perhaps simply by association. Britain was now out of step with numerous other European countries where sodomy was no longer a capital crime: for example, France, Russia, Austria and Prussia; in fact the last execution for sodomy in mainland Europe was in the Dutch Netherlands in 1803. It was of course still a crime, but not one you could lose your life over. There was one moment of respite in Britain however: in 1816 the pillory ceased to be used as a punishment. Moral condemnation of people who loved within their own gender – especially men – continued and even intensified; in the middle of the nineteenth century, visitors who happened upon certain areas or streets in London complained about the large number of ' Margeries and Pooffs' they saw.

Anne Lister

Meanwhile, women could pursue same-sex relationships without fear of arrest (on the whole), but there is rarely so detailed an account than that of the exploits of Anne Lister (1791–1840). In 1826, Lister inherited the West Yorkshire estate of Shibden Hall near Halifax from her uncle, although she had been living there since 1815. Before one examines the writings of Anne Lister, it should be pointed out that Anne came from generations of incumbents of the Shibden estate and as such, was established local gentry. She was literate, unashamedly sapphist, and never married; partly, one could surmise, because of her sexuality, but also perhaps because it would certainly interfere with her independence and freedom to run her estates and her life – and handle her own money – as she saw fit. Despite all this, she still felt the need to write that part of her diary, which included detailed descriptions of her relationships with women, in a cipher so that no-one else could read the intimate details of her exploits. The cipher was made up of a combination of algebra and Ancient Greek, a code that was cracked in the 1980s so that the whole of Anne's life could be revealed. The diaries in total amount to about four million words; she began writing in 1806, continuing until her death in 1840 and writing more as the years went by – approximately half the diary was written in the last decade.

Anne began her diary to record her love for Eliza Raine, whom she met at boarding school in York at the age of 15. It would be all too easy to attribute this relationship to a Freudian model and suggest it was just a 'crush', but bearing in mind Anne's lifetime of Sapphic relationships, it is reasonable to suggest that this was the first of Anne's same-sex loves. The affair with Eliza sadly ended due to the latter's mental health problems, and subsequently Anne went on to have relationships with Isabella Norcliffe ('Tib', from Malton in Yorkshire) and Mariana Belcombe (an affair that continued after Mariana's marriage to Charles Lawton in 1816). By 1821 Anne was so confident of her attractions to women that on 29 January, she wrote in her diary, 'I love and only love the fairer sex and thus, beloved by them in turn, my heart revolts from any other love than theirs'. By 1824 Anne was in Paris, and was pursuing one Mrs Maria Barlow with such success that they eventually found an apartment together, although Anne's lover seems to have been tormented by guilt and some jealousy during the affair. With the diaries we can follow Anne's love life in all its detail (much of it sexual) as well as all the everyday details of the life of a gentlewoman from the provinces. We know that Anne always wore black, that she was seen as noticeably masculine in her mannerisms, had a strong interest in business and running her estate – very much a hands-on manager – and that she contracted a veneral disease, possibly from Mariana via her philandering husband. Anne did not like her women to make love to her, preferring instead to take control in sexual encounters, and was greatly taken aback when Maria Barlow tried to do this, complaining that 'This is womanizing me too much' (19 March 1825), and noting in her diary that Mariana was a much more compatible partner for her as she never tried to take the lead. Anne left Paris at the end of March and left a sorrowful Maria behind, although Anne does seem to be somewhat relieved to be getting away from her.

Anne Lister had a definite advantage over some of her poorer Sapphic sisters, in that she could use her status to conceal her activities or to rise above any public ridicule she faced. In fact, it was necessary to conceal her affairs from the families of some of her lovers, although her own family were uneasily aware of her sapphism and seemed to accept there was little they could do about it. Her social equals regarded her as perhaps a little odd, but were tolerant of her flirtations – after all, she could do no real harm, not being able to give any woman a child. Despite what would now be known as having 'played the field' for years, by the time Anne reached her forties she dearly wished to find a life companion with whom she could settle down. Anne's last relationship was with neighbouring landowner Ann Walker, who was 29 when they met. This was perhaps not the grand passion of Anne's life – she wrote in her diary on 31 August 1832, 'if she was fond of me and manageable, I think I could be comfortable enough with her.' By the beginning of October, Anne was writing of having persuaded Ann to live with her at Shibden Hall and the relationship was deepening: '"… we both probably felt more like lovers than friends …." Thought I, "She's in for it, if ever a girl was – and so am I too."' By December it is clear that there was an established sexual element to their relationship. Apart from the physical side, the affair fulfilled Anne's desire not only to have some emotional stability in her life, but also a chance of advancing her financial status; it took Anne approximately one month to woo Ann and for them to agree that they were in a 'liaison', as Anne put it and it was to mature into a form of covert 'marriage', not just on a personal but on a business level – they were both keen to capitalise on the natural resources on their respective estates and they both re-wrote their wills in favour of each other. Like some of her other romances, the relationship was not without setbacks, notably caused by Ann's religion-based guilt and fears for her fragile health; they were certainly not together all the time, but it was enduring.

Anne comes across as a thoroughly modern woman in many ways. Independent, strong-minded, intent on building her business interests, free to love and be loved as she wished and apparently completely at ease with her sexuality; she lived her life with gusto and wrote compellingly about it with a detail that really draws in the reader and gives a rounded picture of the woman and her life and loves. Elsewhere in this book, comment has been made about the ethical issues around the 'outing' of individuals. In the case of Anne, she never actively concealed her desire for women although at times she was careful to whom she revealed her feelings – she was more circumspect in the less open-minded locality of Halifax, for instance, than in what was, to her, the cosmopolitan society of York. Anne did write of her exploits with women in a cipher for a reason, however. No doubt such details would be deeply shocking if any family read them, or any literate servants who happened to go prying in her private rooms. It may also have been a feeling that she wanted to keep such intimate details for herself, to hold them close as it were, and to make them special; perhaps Anne was a romantic after all! Whatever her reasons, should we now be picking over the deciphered accounts of her intimate relationships? Most historians would say an emphatic yes, as there is so little for us to go by when it comes to genuine, written accounts of the lives of those in same-sex relationships at that time, especially women. We did the same with the diaries of Samuel Pepys, who related with glee his sexual exploits and flirtations, so the precedent is there. In any case, Anne would have been out and proud today and, in a twenty-first century setting, would more than likely have told you anyway, over a glass or two of wine!

The Increasing Regulation of Society

Criminalisation of homosexual acts – as opposed to the crime of committing a single category of sexual act (sodomy) against any person – came in a century when a number of other previously accepted behaviours also became criminalised. During the nineteenth century Britain was taking many, and sometimes painful, steps towards becoming a modern nation; this meant that with increasing industrialisation, a rising population and cultural pressures, there was a perceived need for closer regulation of what people did. Almost alongside the machines of the age, manufacturing identical products by the thousand, was a desire to see people's behaviour homogenised and sanitised. The best way to achieve this was through the application of the law.

From 1 July 1837, registration of life events became a secular process under the remit of a new Registrar General. This was a role that had previously belonged largely to the Anglican Church, and this was the first of many pieces of legislation that reduced the power of the Church, in local life in particular, and pushed the nation into a much more secularised system – poor relief, and most other aspects of local government were removed from the Church. By the end of the century, the Church was reduced mainly to concentrating on its spiritual responsibilities.

In 1857, the Obscene Publications bill was introduced to parliament. Lord Campbell, whose project this was, was campaigning against the growth of pornographic publications, which he regarded as more dangerous than the sale of poisons such as prussic acid (a substance that was mentioned again in connection with the novel *The Well of Loneliness* in 1928; see below). Once the act was passed, pretty much any disorderly or immoral behaviour was an offence, including swearing, drunkenness, and other 'dissolute, immoral, or disorderly practices' – an impossibly broad remit for law enforcers but a gift for the narrow minded. Obscene or indecent publications could now be seized and destroyed, making their publications a much more serious offence than the common law misdemeanour it previously was. From the very beginning the act was open to wide interpretation, and following a ruling in 1868 in the case *Regina v Hicklin*, any printed work with anything approaching sexual content that it was thought could 'deprave and corrupt' fell on the wrong side of the law. This 'Hicklin Test' would prove particularly useful when 'moralistic' campaigners wanted to target any publication with even the vaguest of same-sex content.

In 1861, the Offences Against the Person Act formally abolished the death penalty for buggery in England and Wales. It should be remembered that sodomy, or buggery, was an offence whether the gender mix of the two participants was male–male, or male–female, and as a result, anyone could be accused, although it was generally the male–male associations that attracted the closest attention of the law

Public order offences and gambling became subject to legislation – gambling was a victim of the moral disapproval of the habit. Poaching became theft, and no doubt many a 'weekend' poacher looking for some fresh meat for the family pot fell foul of a law he did not even know was in place. Some sporting activities came under the scrutiny of the law, and were more frequently oppressed by legal means if it was deemed to be disturbing the peace, or perhaps more importantly, trade. Boisterous or loud public celebrations also suffered in the same way; the 1875 Explosives Act, Section 80 prohibited 'the setting off of fireworks on any highway, street, thoroughfare or public place'.

CHAPTER TWO

Alcohol was increasingly regulated; from 1869 beer houses had to be licensed, and a further Licensing Act in 1872 gave Justices of the Peace control of all beer houses, virtually bringing to an end the informal selling of alcohol. The sale of another foodstuff – milk – was regulated to reduce the risk of tuberculosis, and the 1869 the Contagious Diseases (Animals) Act brought a farmer's animals within the remit of the law if they contracted a disease such as foot and mouth.

In public health, the Vaccination Acts of 1840, 1853, 1867 and 1898 were a step towards better child welfare and public health improvements, and the 1851 Common Lodging Houses Act was one of a series of steps taken to regulate areas thought to be a health risk.

Even worship was scrutinised – in 1840 the Church Discipline Act was passed relating to the behaviour of clerics, and the 1874 Public Worship Regulation Act aimed to prevent ritualistic worship in the Church of England.

It is therefore no surprise that the attention of the law was also directed to the sexual behaviour of the population, and in particular, their expression of sexuality.

In 1885, the Criminal Law Amendment Act was passed. Essentially this was a useful piece of legislation designed primarily to protect young girls; for example, it raised the age of consent for girls from 13 to 16 years old. However, it was also to become the weapon by which men who were found to be in a compromising situation with another male were prosecuted, some might say persecuted. It was this very act that, about a decade later, was to bring about the downfall of Oscar Wilde. Many amendments were suggested for the bill, but one eventually became part of the act, making full use of the words 'other purposes' at the end of the subtitle (see list of sources) – the Labouchere Amendment. Henry Labouchere was a Liberal and one of the members of parliament for Northampton and on 6 August he introduced the following:

Any male person who, in public or private, commits, or is a party to the commission of, or procures, or attempts to procure the commission by any male person of, any act of gross indecency with another male person, shall be guilty of a misdemeanour, and being convicted thereof, shall be liable at the discretion of the Court to be imprisoned for any term not exceeding two years, with or without hard labour.

No reference in the act is made to women with same-sex desires who acted upon them. A total of 8,921 men had been prosecuted since 1806 for sodomy, with 404 sentenced to death and fifty-six executed. Now the new threat to men who loved within their own sex was a law that was not so easy to circumvent, and still threatened public humiliation in court and a gruelling spell in prison, with the subsequent struggle on release of finding a new life and work for themselves, sometimes without the support of their family. Rather like the Hicklin Test, the notion of gross indecency is not explained and pretty much left to the imaginations of the prosecutors. Presumably, if felt to be arousing enough, any sexual or intimate activity between men could qualify, and whilst sodomy was left as a separate serious offence, many men who may have escaped the wrath of the law before this act could now fall into its clutches. If matters did not get that far, these men were highly susceptible to blackmail, and in fact the act became known as the 'blackmailer's charter' as most men duped by blackmailers would pay up rather than face court and gaol. It is not surprising also that there are some accounts of men in prison being prosecuted for 'unnatural crimes', as happened in 1853 with William Hodson who was accused of trying to commit an unnatural crime with a fellow prisoner in Dartmoor Prison. Hodson was sentenced to two extra years in prison on top of his ten-year sentence for robbery, which had begun in 1850. He subsequently received a pardon for the two-year sentence, with no reason being given.

The strictures of this huge swathe of acts of parliament was ineffective if not observed, of course, and the establishment had an advantage in that the new police forces around the country were not only the ideal monitors of potential miscreants, but were also ideally placed to apply the law as required. Although the primary and avowed role of the new police forces was the prevention of crime, they did respond to many an incident where new laws were broken, whether out of ignorance or wilfully. However, no amount of legislation is going to prevent many people doing what they want to do, or are drawn to do; it simply pushed the activity into the covert, where secrecy and silence are the watchwords.

An unexpected advantage for the public at the time – and for historians subsequently – is that extra legislation meant more contraventions, and that meant newsworthy stories. Add to this the rapid growth of the provincial newspapers in the nineteenth century and greater literacy with which to enjoy them, and there is a ready market eager for scandal –

CHAPTER TWO

tabloid-style reporting with lurid illustrations dominated publications such as the *Illustrated Police News*, whilst the upmarket newspapers such as *The Times* and *Manchester Guardian* took the moral high ground with serious, sermon-like editorials. As historian Florence Tamagne states: '... it was scandal that frequently brought homosexuality to the attention of the public at large, notably through the workings of the new mass media. By means of a skilful mixture of facts and accounts of 'perversions', newspapers sought to capture the minds of their volatile readers.' It was a crushing blow to any person involved in same-sex relationships, be they sodomite or sapphist, to be humiliated and exposed in the newspapers, but had this not happened, unless they had ended up in court, we more than likely would have nothing about them, their lives or their relationships. The historian gains knowledge, it could be said, at the expense of those who felt pain and humiliation at the time.

Romantic Friendships Between Victorian Women

One aspect of women-oriented life was the prevalence of strong, sometimes romantically-inclined all female relationships, something that had echoes in the close friendships of women in the previous century. In some middle-class circles, such intimate friendships were, if not encouraged, certainly accepted, as it was much safer for a married woman to have a passionate friendship with another woman than to even contemplate a close friendship with a man other than her husband. With contraceptive advice in short supply and even when used, not universally successful, a woman in an illicit affair with a man risked an inappropriate pregnancy, and thus separation and even divorce for the wealthy and almost certainly alienation from her children who, if only for strictly economic and security reasons, would stay with their father. This is not to say that men did not, knowingly or unknowingly, raise children that were not their own; but if a middle-class man did this, he risked the other male coming forward, claiming the child was his, and trying to stake a claim on the family finances and inheritance. In 1857, the Matrimonial Causes Act made it easier for more people to divorce, and stripped away the confusing system that had been in place before; it also took away from the Church yet more power in an important area. Because it was easier for a husband to obtain a divorce than for a wife, it was therefore much 'safer' all round for a woman who spent much of her time in a female dominated sphere – the home – to build a strong bond with another woman.

This friendship could take the form of writing fond letters, sending poems to each other, and offering mutual support and affection in varying degrees, and historians can interpret these surviving letters, diaries and other writings as evidence that a close bond existed. As for the physical side of that friendship, that was a much more private matter, but there is evidence of hand-holding, kissing, and fondling. There may well have been more, but propriety – and a need to keep such strong passions discreet – meant these moments are rarely recorded.

In working-class families there was no time – or education – to indulge in poetry or hand-holding. Instead, support and affection would have been snatched between heavy household work and intimacy may have been guarded in a small two or four roomed house with children running in and out, and menfolk and older daughters coming home at odd times from shift work. How could these women express their feelings for the neighbour who was there for them no matter what? Passionate attachments may well have been seen by family as just mother asking 'Aunty Bessie from next door' for a bit of help on a regular basis or calling round to see her for a cup of tea if there was time. For some women, that intimacy would have been in the childbirth room, with men excluded; there can be few more intimate moments than witnessing a woman you are close to give birth. No doubt the bonds forged at those moments would have intensified any friendship. Where there is affection, the parties involved will find a way of expressing those feelings.

Are these friendships what we would now see as lesbian relationships? Some feminist writers would say they are, and in fact would say they are the purest form of female same-sex relationships and that all lesbian romances are as pure as this. The sentiments echo what Oscar Wilde said in his trial later in the century – that a love between two people of the same sex could be as pure and unblemished as any other, if not more so. Often these women did not live in the same household; sometimes the friendship might be with a woman in the extended family – the American poet Emily Dickinson was passionately attached to her sister-in-law, Sue Gilbert. We might now call them 'best friends' or lifelong friends, but it still remains a same-sex relationship that was usually enduring (menfolk permitting), loyal, deeply loving and often passionate, if only on a romantic level. When fear of inevitable and often dangerous childbirth followed a marriage – even if precautions were taken, it was expected that there would be some children from that marriage – it is little wonder that women sought each other out for emotional support and practical help, and possibly, a freedom of intimacy that would not result in yet another unwanted pregnancy.

Sometimes, however, there is more reason than not to assume a sexual relationship between two women. Emily Faithfull (1835–1895) was a pioneer in the promotion of employment for women, and amongst other achievements opened the Victoria Press with a largely female workforce in 1860. Probably because they were worried at this innovation of female compositors, the trade unions protested, claiming that having men and women working together in a print shop (the men were there to do the heavy work) would lead to immoral goings-on. Nevertheless, the Victoria Press was a success, not only commercially, but in the high standards it set for good working conditions for employees. In 1864, however, Emily was involved as the third party in scandalous divorce case between Admiral Henry Codrington and his wife, Helen Jane. Emily and Helen had begun a love affair in 1854, whilst the Admiral was deployed abroad in the Crimean War. He returned home two years later to find Emily had usurped his place in Helen's bed and worse still, Helen was refusing to be a 'proper' wife to him. His Victorian patriarchal sensibilities enraged, the Admiral threw Emily out of his house and deposited with his brother a packet of incriminating paperwork, possibly letters between the two women. Emily was called as a witness in the divorce case, but the scandal did not seem to damage her illustrious career as a campaigner and speaker on, and for, women's matters, working tirelessly to improve the lives of dressmakers, cotton operatives, and women who had fallen on hard times. In 1892, she even received a Civil List pension of £50 per year and a signed photograph of Queen Victoria.

At about the same time as society was dividing the workplace and domestic life into two distinctly separate spheres, a greater definition was growing over what was acceptable masculine and feminine behaviour. The Victorian ideal of manliness was growing in favour, to the detriment of men who were less masculine or – heaven forbid – positively effeminate. Women and girls were expected to adhere strictly to the middle-class precept of being demure, obedient, domestic and gentle, even though most working-class females lived lives of unrelenting toil, either at home or in domestic service, agriculture or industry. This is not to say that men could not be gentle – a saintly self sacrifice was acceptable, especially if in the name of honour or family, but if they were men who were to go out into the world and create and govern, then their softer side had to be shown in strict moderation. In addition, a real man was capable of practicing sexual continence – purity – and any man who was promiscuous, even with women, was frowned upon; restraint was the order of the day. Thus, at about the same time as men and women were being separated into distinct areas of activity, masculine men and effeminate men were also being categorised.

In addition, the idea that artistic pursuits, as a 'soft' non-commercial activity, were essentially feminine was taking hold. If one therefore puts together that effeminacy was to be kept separate from masculine behaviour, and aligns an interest in the arts with women too, one gets a correlation between effeminate men and the arts which was to prevail as a stereotypical view of homosexual men for many years, and was reinforced in the minds of the public during and after the trials of Oscar Wilde.

Case Study: Three Female Husbands of Manchester

Harry Stokes

Meanwhile, far away from the genteel middle-class parlours of the new suburbs and the hand-holding passionate female friends, in the smoke and grit of industrial Manchester in 1859, a sad death occurred. Henry or Harry Stokes, respected bricklayer, special constable and a man who had worked on some of the proud city's prestigious new buildings, was found dead in the canal at Pendleton. The evening before he had sat, low in spirits, in the Swan public house and had four glasses of beer, then left, never to be seen alive again, despite saying to staff he was on his way to the Throstle Nest, presumably for another drink. His body was pulled from the water and the inquest would have proceeded to a swift conclusion had not one of the jury recognised Henry as a person who had been embroiled in an extraordinary scandal years before. The coroner instructed two women to examine the body to see if the juror's hunch was correct, and indeed it was; Henry Stokes was found to be a woman, 'full breasted, but the shape of her womanly make was distorted by a broad strap which was buckled round her body under the arms'

(*Liverpool Mercury*, 24 October 1859), and those present realised they were dealing with the death of none other than Harriet 'Henry' Stokes, noted 'female husband' of Manchester who had hit the headlines more than once in the past.

From the outset, some posthumous reports of Stokes's life were sympathetic, even stating that once Stokes had adopted the masculine persona, they 'must drop the female appellative' and refer to Stokes as male from that point on in their narrative. We are told that for thirty years – taking us back to the 1820s – Stokes had:

> *lived in Manchester and Salford as a journeyman and master bricksetter; had twice been married to other women; had kept beerhouses and served customers at the tap as a 'jolly land-lord'; had worked her trade as a bricksetter and erected many important buildings in both towns; and had obtained the rep-utation of being the most skilful fire-grate setter and 'chimney doctor' in the neighbourhood. She always dressed as a man, in the clothing peculiar to her trade; invariably superintended the men in her employment; and could lift a weight, spread the mortar, and set a brick with the best of them.*
> *(Liverpool Mercury,* 24 October 1859*)*

The unwitting male population of the two cities were also to find out that they had accepted Stokes as one of their own in their drinking places, where she 'drank, smoked, and joked with the hardest, and joined in the evening carousals.'

In fact, compared to the female husbands in the rest of this case study, the life of Harry Stokes is pretty straightforward to put together from a variety of sources, and the fact that she came under the scrutiny of the law more than once is a big help as details had to be taken down and kept on record – and a brush with the law often made it to the newspapers too. We get to know Harry through an astonishing range of sources including the census, newspapers, parish registers, rate books and trade directories. From the various reports and census returns we learn that Harry (as we will refer to her from now on, as that is what she used informally), was born in the Doncaster area in about 1799, apparently the daughter of a bricklayer. Life was hard at home and there are hints of violence in the family, which caused Harry to run away at the age of 8, dressed in boys' clothes; Harry ended up as working for a bricklayer to whom she was later apprenticed. It should be noted here that for a child to be working hard at the age of 8 was not uncommon at the turn of the nineteenth century, and this does have the ring of truth about it.

We next meet Harry in her teens, when she seems to have got married in the Cathedral Church of St Peter and St Paul, Sheffield on 14 January 1817. The bride is one Ann Hants; an unusual surname, but the name Hant is not unknown in Yorkshire and even if not her own, it is not a 'made-up' surname. There is a curious mistake on the marriage entry, which shows that not only did Harry and her wife both have literacy skills – no crosses instead of names here – but that Harry almost wrote her real name – Harriet – and then crossed it out. That must have been a moment of panic for her! Although the surname is spelt differently – here it is Stoake, a known variant of the surname Stoke(s) – it is reasonable to accept this as Harry's own marriage.

Newspaper reports tell us that the couple moved to Manchester some time after that, and certainly by the mid 1820s Harry is advertising in the trade directories as a bricklayer 'and by considerable skill, ability, and attention to trade, was tolerably successful … this builder became remarkable, indeed, almost to celebrity, for skill and success in the erection of flues, ovens etc' (*Sheffield Independent* 14 April 1838). Harry was so successful that she became an employer, and Ann (assuming she had the same wife then) dealt with the accounts. Rates books, beautifully completed in copperplate handwriting, show us Harry and Ann's various addresses at this period in their lives; not the best of areas, but perhaps they felt their relationship would be safe enough in a district where their neighbours were unlikely to report any suspicions to the authorities lest their own crimes and misdemeanours be found out. All seemed to be going well until marital turmoil threatened Harry's cover, relationship, and identity, and revealed her secret to the world; her wife went to a lawyer, Mr Thomas, and complained that Harry was withholding her housekeeping money, and generally treating her unkindly, and then revealed to the astonished lawyer that her husband was, in fact, female. How should she proceed in obtaining redress when her partner was in fact of the same gender as her? The bemused lawyer decided to consult the magistrate, Mr Foster, who suggested that both parties be brought before him at the police office to be questioned. Harry had to undergo the indignity of a physical examination by Mr Ollier, the police surgeon, who confirmed Ann's story. Ann added to her grievances by stating that Harry was sometimes drunk and that she in turn had been very loyal to Harry *after discovering three years before that Harry was in fact female,* in other words, eighteen years into the marriage!

From the report in the *Sheffield Independent* (14 April 1838) it would appear that the couple had separated, as Harry sent some of Ann's possessions to the police office, presumably for her to collect, and it would seem that shortly afterwards, Mr Thomas managed to persuade Harry to let Ann have their house and contents, in lieu of the maintenance that a 'real' husband would have given his wife and as acknowledgement for all Ann's support of Harry's business over the years, and for keeping house for them both. It is unlikely that Mr Thomas ever thought he would end up as mediator and counsellor to an all female couple with relationship problems! The newspaper also stated that word had got around about Harry's true identity and:

> *… the woman who has ventured to assume the character of a man will no longer be able to continue to carry on business in this town* [Manchester], *and that she must either lay aside her disguise, or resume the appearance that most befits her sex; or, is she will retain her unfeminine appearance and character, she must seek to hide her imposture in some place where she is not known.*

How wrong that reporter was. Harry carried on regardless, although she does seem to have withdrawn from her role as special constable at about this time, whether because of the fact that she had a raised visibility with the public, or because marital problems had distracted her, it is impossible to say. After Harry's death, a syndicated biography from the *Salford Weekly News,* which circulated around many provincial newspapers, tells the tale of a new wife for Harry, named Betsy, who seems to have been the next potentially long-term partner. Betsy apparently was a 'plump little widow' who kept a beer house in Cupid's Alley off what is now a prestige shopping area in Manchester, but which was then not a smart area to be in at all. We are told that 'He had been accustomed to take his pot of beer and smoke his short pipe under Betsy's roof and had at least taken a decided fancy to Betsy herself.' They married, but it all went wrong on the wedding night when Harry was revealed as female: 'The night was spent in downright quarrel and fight; and the lamentable result was a summons taken out by Betsy against her husband for assault, for which he was condemned to the New Bailey for one or two months.' Betsy declared forcefully to the court that she had no idea her new husband was a woman and she certainly was not going to live with Harry – clearly Harry had made a serious error of judgement in choosing Betsy as a spouse. Not only did Harry lose her bride, she also became the butt of popular jokes and street ballads, was tormented by street urchins and teased by workmates. Harry stood firm, hinting that Betsy was a little bit mad to suggest such a thing and refusing to discuss her own gender with anyone.

At some point after that, Harry met and married her last wife, a widow somewhat older than her named Frances Collins. She had grown-up children who came to look upon Harry as a doting father, they were together for as long as Harry and Ann were, and yet Frances claimed after she was widowed a second time that she had had no idea that Harry was female. She also claimed that she took Harry in because she felt sorry for her, but if she felt sorry for her because of what had happened to her, then she certainly knew with whom she was co-habiting.

The Liverpool Mercury also expressed surprise that Harry had managed all those years 'having throughout the whole of her remarkable life maintained a remarkable check upon those passions which crowd the streets of every large town with the unfortunate of her sex'; in other words, she did a remarkable job of keeping her feelings for men under control, especially in view of the fact that she was with men both at work and socially, and in close quarters! The Victorian reader must have wondered about those repressed female passions, metaphorically strapped down along with Harry's breasts. There is no hint here that Stokes was unhappy in her choice of female partners and yet the newspapers imply that she chose women lovers because she dare not go looking for a man; the fact that some women insisted that they never knew their female husbands were in fact women, also supports the preconception that the arrangement was purely domestic and not romantic or sexual, and that a woman partner was a pragmatic choice rather than a romantic one. This all fits in with the Victorian notion of the passive and sexless women who had no interest in sexual passion and therefore two such women, as in a passionate middle-class female–female friendship, were more than likely celibate.

CHAPTER TWO

Ann McGaul/John Jones

Another woman was seemingly the antithesis of feminine wiles. In early spring 1862, one Ann McGaul, alias Ann Hughes, alias John Jones, was standing in front of the city magistrates charged with (as the *Dundee Courier* of 29 March put it) 'annoying the landlady of a lodging house … by creating a disturbance and threatening to beat another woman named Sarah Jones, with whom the prisoner had been living as husband.' Ann, or John, had been passing as male for six years, so that she could earn the higher wages of a man – 2/6d per week instead the woman's wage of a shilling a week. At one point she had worked as a banksman in a colliery (a surface job with responsibility for the cage and winding gear that transported colliers down the shaft). One awkward time in Ann's life passing as a man was the four nights she had to sleep in the same bed as the landlady's son due to lack of space in the lodging house or 'establishment' as the newspaper wryly calls it (implying that it was a brothel; in fact many brothels appear as 'lodging houses' or similar on census returns) and was never found out. Standing in the dock, Ann/John claimed she had no other clothes than the masculine ones they saw her in, and originally came from Gillmoss, which is in north Liverpool. She was discharged, having promised not to repeat the annoyance to the landlady, but had to wait for a while in the courtroom as a crowd had assembled outside and the authorities feared she would be mobbed on leaving – whether the crowd was hostile or just plain boisterous and curious, it does not say.

Thomas Green

Only a few months later, one Thomas Green was allowed to walk free from court in Salford after another apprehension in connection with non-payment of debt, the debt in question being for a suit of men's clothes. Green objected strongly to yet another spell in gaol but Judge Trafford was insistent, and ordered that the prisoner bathe before going to his cell to see if it would moderate his temper. On being forced to undress, prison officers found to their astonishment that Green was in fact female, and in a happy 'marriage' to another woman. Green thought she had a plausible explanation for passing as male. She said that as a girl, she had been employed by a lady who really wanted a page, not a maid, and Green had therefore been dressed in boy's clothes to satisfy her whim. The habit stuck, and Green grew up continuing to dress in male attire, with the advantage of earning a man's wage – at one point working in a mill as a hooker and stitcher. Apparently comfortably off but lonely, Green had then looked for a woman to share her life with. We are told that Green, 'after a curious interrogation, was dismissed to her affectionate wife.' (*The Times*, 7 May 1861).

Cases like the latter two here are a real conundrum for the researcher. Any person who adopts aliases probably has more of them than they actually say (and would find it no bother at all to concoct more if needed), and it is extremely difficult to ascertain which is real, and then corroborate it, as these individuals are often estranged from family too. In this sense they are rather like the petty criminals of the day, constantly looking for a persona to conceal their real identity, the fear of discovery ever present. Names could be 'borrowed' from chance acquaintances, friends, or something read in a newspaper or overheard in a public house. Someone like Ann McGaul may have to leave the area, at least for a time, to let things calm down a bit, and the chances are a new alias would be created for the simple purpose of self preservation, to aid the chances of getting a job, and simply to ensure some peace and quiet. In this sense, passing women could find themselves living a similar life to a petty thief, moving around to avoid people getting to know them too well, keeping a low profile from the authorities, but still needing the emotional and practical security of a home and spouse. Because of their name changes, the spellings of the names we know about can be more volatile than usual too. As an example, if one looks for Ann McGaul/John Jones in the census returns, she is nowhere to be seen. Attempts to find an Ann McGaul or an Ann Hughes in baptism registers in the area of Liverpool she claimed to be from – Gillmoss – have proved so far unsuccessful. We don't even know if she is telling the truth about any of her names, and the choice of Jones as a very common surname was clever – if she had adopted her wife's surname she would have known it would offer some anonymity, as the large Welsh migrant population in her native Liverpool would have shown her.

Looking at the census returns for 1861, Ann is difficult to locate. However, if you broaden the search to Lancashire, an interesting possibility comes up. At Bowker Fold, Kearsley, lived a John and Sarah Jones. John was born in 1834, and Sarah in 1843, and with them is a lodger, Gervase

CHAPTER TWO

Tarbuck, 36 years old and born in Euxton, about eighteen miles away. Kearsley was an industrialised area by this time and had well in excess of a dozen collieries that John/Ann could have worked at. However, at the same time in a lodging house in Pigeon Street, Manchester, there is an Ann McGill, not so far a leap from the original name she claimed to have – and lodging-house keepers were notoriously bad at getting the details of their lodgers right on the census. There is also a 15-year-old boy there, the son of the landlady, and he could well be the boy that Ann bunked in with when beds were short in 1862. There is a Sarah, but she is a child and does not fit the criteria to be anyone's spouse. Is this our female husband in 1861? We don't know if she even had a partner that year, and much more extensive work must be done to uncover the truth, if that is at all possible. Until more facts are uncovered *and verified*, we must leave Ann in her lodging house in 1862, with her aliases and her turbulent lifestyle.

Bearing in mind the problems that can accompany research into those who passed as the other gender, we are very fortunate in that Harriet Stokes seemed to have an innate honesty – or courage – in going by a name as close to her own as possible. It is but a small jump from Harriet Stokes to Harry or Henry Stokes, and so confident was she of acceptance as Henry that she fully involved herself in public life, and stuck doggedly to her constructed identity even in the face of public taunting and humiliation, to the point where even the newspapers spoke admiringly of her courage at all levels. One wonders how crucified with humiliation she would have been had she known her body would have been stripped bare – literally – and chattered about in a public courtroom and beyond, with newspaper reports that detailed her full figure and the large breasts that she tried so hard to conceal. Harriet strove hard to make a living for herself and her wives, and it would seem she craved respectability too, taking the risk of putting herself in public life in order to make her mark on her adopted town.

The issue of gender needs to be addressed here too. How are we to think of these women, who lived in an age when few labels existed for females who lived these extraordinary lives? All three of these women – and no doubt many others who lived and died incognito, living in plain sight of their unsuspecting neighbours – passed as male for years, if not a lifetime. Should we therefore label them as transgendered and as people who would, if alive today, assign themselves as heterosexual males, in view of the fact that they lived in happy marriages, which to the outside world looked like a man and a woman? Are their 'wives' lesbian, or are they simply women who looked for someone to care for them and who wouldn't drive them into poverty with a houseful of babies, surely an advantage to a poor woman? Frances Collins, the last wife of Harry Stokes, claimed she took Harry in because she felt sorry for her and went along with the relationship in order to save Harry from the constant ridicule she suffered – to show people that Harry was actually a husband in all but gender. Surely, gender and sexuality are more complex than simplistic labelling. Today, passing women, cross-dressing women, or whatever label you choose to give them, have every opportunity to self-identify with a number of 'labels', and this gives them some visibility in a society that likes everyone to slot into a pigeon hole. Harry and her 'brothers' had no such luxury and no doubt if you asked them to identify as anything, may well have answered that they were just trying to get by, that they fell in love with women and not men (and may not even have questioned this within themselves), and that they just wanted anonymity in which to live their lives in peace. As to why they dressed as men, the vast majority of female husbands told remarkably similar tales of having to leave home or employment at a young age, and dress as boys in order to get by and be safe out there in the world alone. This may be only part of the truth; Judith Halberstam sees masculinity in women as a much more complex characteristic than we think, so the inner need of these women to present as male is difficult to quantify in a few sentences. Poet and academic Minnie Bruce Pratt once described her transgendered partner as her 'lesbian husband' and this is a phrase that seems to suit our Victorian women very well whether they had gender 'issues' or not. Transgendered, lesbian, or otherwise, these unique same-sex relationships are a constant fascination to the modern researcher, just as they were to the eager newspaper readers of the past.

One aspect of these 'female husband' stories which crops up regularly is the statements by the wives or partners that they knew nothing of the gender of their 'husband' until either the wedding night, or a point some time after the marriage was established. In some cases this might have been a pre-arranged course of action in the event of exposure to protect the spouses from public condemnation as freaks or as less than women themselves, a strategy born out of the female husband's love for their wife; Ann Stokes only revealed Harry's secret during a marital dispute and presumably would have kept quiet otherwise. Thomas Green was lucky in that the wife in this partnership was out and proud about her spouse, making no secret of it.

Finally, the tone of the newspaper articles is worthy of mention. There is certainly a respect and affection for Harry Stokes, which does not seem to be tongue-in-cheek, as the closing words of one article show:

> *There is something of grandeur, after all, in the character of that strange woman. She has left mementoes of her industry and skill all over Manchester, and in many places in Salford. She was very clever in the erection of tall chimneys … she has built churches, chapels, and extensive blocks of dwelling houses … she was most expert in fitting stoves and firegrates … in some of the best houses in Manchester, and in the days of the Chartist riots … was made captain of her company* [of special constables].

Harry's reputation was saved at the end because she had helped to make her adopted city even greater, and civic pride was assuaged.

Men Passing as Women: Fanny and Stella

In 1870 and 1871, Thomas Ernest Boulton ('Stella', 1847–1904) and Frederick William Park ('Fanny', 1846–1881), both from middle-class families, stood trial for conspiring and inciting persons to commit an unnatural offence, along with six associates. They appeared in court in full female garb, their defence claiming that they cross-dressed for a lark and did not do so to entice gentlemen to their apartments to extort money from them, and any 'perverted' correspondence they received from other males was plain foolishness on their part and not encouraged. The Defence Counsel described one of the men as a 'dainty and pleasing boy' and hinted that it was no wonder some other men should get carried away by their beauty. The jury acquitted the accused after less than an hour's deliberation, and some in the press suggested that the whole case had been a waste of time. These young men, who made extremely attractive women in their carefully constructed outfits with female shaping, wigs and accessories and had been cross-dressing from a young age, were brazen, unrepentant and coquettish, and yet everyone seemed to suggest that these boys were just pranksters and should have been left alone! It may be that Fanny and Stella were lucky to have been tried when they were, at a time when homosexuality as an illness or perversion was a notion that was extremely new and had not begun to circulate outside some rarified academic circles; had they been arrested at the time Oscar Wilde was later in the century, the outcome could have been very different. What seemed to upset people more than their sexual preferences, was the fact that they were cross-dressing and thereby duping some, but by no means all, of their male acquaintances; many of the men who associated with Fanny and Stella were well aware of the gender of the objects of their admiration. So appealing were Fanny and Stella as women that they had a successful career on the stage as entertainers, and a letter written in their defence during the trial in 1870 described an amateur performance the two had given in Essex in which: 'Their admirable acting and marvellous make-up created the greatest excitement and enthusiasm ... bouquets were thrown to them on the stage, supper parties were given at gentlemen's houses, at which they were specially requested to appear in female attire.' (*London Evening Standard* 10 May 1870). A number of men wrote admiring and rather compromising letters to Fanny and Stella, and there is little doubt that they had same-sex relationships even though this was not proven in court. The heyday of Fanny and Stella coincided perfectly with the labelling of same-sex desire as an illness, but they were flamboyant and lucky enough to escape the onslaught of the mind doctors.

The Medicalisation of Same-Sex Desires

Leaving aside the law regarding sodomy, the nineteenth century is highly significant for the transition from same-sex relationships as an immoral act to the medicalisation of men and women who desired their own gender as patients, lunatics, or freaks of nature. Ambroise Tardieu (1818–1878) wrote *Medico-Legal Study of Indecent Assaults* (1857), in which there was one chapter about relations between men. Although the study was largely designed to aid the courts in identifying signs of sodomy in the male physique, it still represents a growing interest on the part of the maturing medical profession, a profession that was looking to consolidate a monopoly on all matters relating to the human body, its ailments and cures. The detail with which Tardieu outlines his study is eerily reminiscent of the witch hunts of previous centuries, which offered advice on how to recognise a witch via physical signs – he compiled a list of 'signs of pederasty', which includes use of cosmetics, ostentatious clothes, and lack of personal care, and he is one of the first to point out a difference between the passive and the active partner, which he claimed could be determined from physiological features.

The word *homosexual* was 'invented' in 1868 by Karl Maria Kertbeny, a campaigner against laws in Prussia that criminalised men who had relations with men. In 1869, Kertbeny used the word in a pamphlet published anonymously as part of his campaign – the first time the word was used in print. It has proved both a useful label and a millstone to those who identify with it, and a misleading descriptive for those who are not 'homosexuals'. The word literally means a person who is romantically or sexually attracted to another person of the same gender, 'homo' from the Greek meaning 'same' and 'sexual' from the Medieval Latin *sexualis*. In other words, it is a one-word way of describing same-sex attraction. The difficulty comes with the subliminal message in the word – homo*sex*ual – the word sex stuck right in the midst of what was meant to be a serious label for a newly discovered 'illness' subconsciously suggests that people who experience same gender attraction are dominated by sexual feelings when, as we have already seen, this is simply not always the case. No wonder Oscar Wilde made such a play of romantic attachment within one gender, even leaving aside the serious criminal charges he faced. Wilde simply did not want to be seen as any kind of sexual deviant or predatory sodomitic maniac.

Other terms were also being used alongside homosexual – referring to someone who felt same-sex attraction as an 'invert' was probably more heavily used at that time. Other phrases – 'the third sex', 'contrary sexual feeling' and 'the intermediate sex' were all coined around this time. Clearly though, as time went on, *homosexual* became the word most frequently used by the medical and scientific community to denote those who felt same-sex attraction, and more labels were added to a wide range of people (see below).

This identification of people with same-sex desires as 'homosexual' – flawed as it was for a long time – has been regarded in two ways. One group of academics has seen it as the 'discovery' and labelling of a type of person who has been there throughout history, anonymous because there was no label for them; the second group of researchers sees it as the starting point for the creation of an identity that was never there – of course same-sex relationships appear throughout history, but never in the same context as the next epoch and always regarded differently. Sexual acts that transgressed moral and religious boundaries, such as sodomy, were seen as separate from the person who did them. From the nineteenth century onwards, the person and the act were indissolubly bound together and if one aspect of the person was frowned upon, by default the whole person was flawed. In the mid-nineteenth century, a name and a set of behaviours was imposed upon people with same-sex attractions, and it became something to be analysed, picked over, treated and if necessary, cured. One other unforeseen consequence of this labelling was that as time went by, everyone else acquired labels too. 'Normal' people who fell in love with an opposite gender partner became 'heterosexual'; those who could equally be attracted to either gender (taking gender in simplistic terms) became 'bisexual'. Given time, every human being ended up with a label of some kind, and subsequently, a set of behaviours that was imposed upon them and to which they might have felt compelled to adhere, and if they did not, they were regarded as transgressive.

The theories came thick and fast. In 1864, Karl Heinrich Ulrichs outlined his theory that a homosexual male was essentially a female soul in a man's body; a female homosexual was the reverse, making these people so different as to be a third sex. Ulrichs claimed that the 'condition' was the result of an abnormal development of the brain, and in 1862, coined the word 'urning' (or Uranian, a Greek term for a third sex) for men with a completely normal male body, but a desire to share that body with other men whilst having an aversion to women. He did however argue that homosexuality was a trait that a person was born with, and that it was innate and could not be changed or done away with. Ulrichs was a indefatigable campaigner for equal rights for the newly named Uranian, and he attempted to explain through historical research that same-sex desire was natural, using examples such as the relationship between the Roman Emperor Hadrian and the younger man, Antinous. Austrian academic Richard von-Krafft-Ebing disagreed. He saw homosexuality as a degenerative disorder and a fetish, and highlighted what he saw as mental health weaknesses in the families of those homosexuals he studied. Havelock Ellis, a British sexologist, was one of the first to write a study of the subject that aimed to be completely non judgemental. *Sexual Inversion* had a rocky start to its publishing life, as it was banned after the Oscar Wilde trials, but it was ground breaking in that Ellis was adamant

CHAPTER TWO

that homosexuality was inborn and indeed could be inherited; also, he did not insist that homosexual men and women had perforce to be 'inverted' in their gender behaviours or presentation. Bearing in mind that this was a new science, one must be tolerant of the stranger statements made by the likes of Ellis – he said, for instance, that green was the favourite colour of inverts, that inverts all had child-like faces and that any woman could be seduced by an experienced female invert. Clearly at this time, homosexuality was seen as some form of inbuilt 'deformity', and as such there was little that could be done about it, but it is not a very flattering definition compared to a popular opinion in the late twentieth century that sexuality is like eye colour: it is what it is, and is just another facet of that person's inborn characteristics.

As well as increasing state intervention in people's lives and the pushing of individuals into compartments when it came to sexuality, the way we lived and worked was changing too. More and more people achieved economic independence by engaging in waged labour, often in the newly industrialised processes; in turn, this gave some the freedom to move around for work, aided by the new transport opportunities offered by the railways from the 1830s. Space away from the prying eyes of family and the loose tongues of neighbours may have encouraged some to look for partners who would have been frowned upon in their own locality. This growth in opportunities would have applied to some women too, although the wages in such work as domestic service – which employed 1,237,149 people in 1871, and the restrictions of living in another person's household, would not have helped. Professional women, who increasingly had access to education and training as the century drew to a close, were more able to forge the sort of relationships they wanted. It may or may not be true that homosexual women were drawn to professions such as nursing, for example, because of the all female environment and the 'live-in' accommodation – we will never have any accurate statistics on this – but it must have been tempting if opportunities were lacking in any other way, if only to enjoy a female-oriented environment. In addition, staying single in the pursuit of one's vocation, be that teaching, nursing or any other role, would be seen as selfless and committed, giving some women the opportunity to stay single and not weigh themselves down with the hypocrisy of a marriage that was not wanted, yet displaying those nurturing characteristics that were so prized by the Victorian patriarchy.

The possibilities for women to form bonds in the workplace or predominantly female environments had not escaped the 'experts', either. Famous professor of medicine Thomas Laycock, in his *Treatise on the Nervous Disorders of Women* (1840), expounded his theory that working-class women were especially prone to abnormal attachments:

> *Hysteria is often seen amongst semptresses, lace-workers, and other of the female population of large towns, confined for many hours daily at sedentary employments, or in heated manufacto-ries; and who, from associating in numbers, excite each other's passions.*

Whilst Laycock may be predominantly referring to mental health abnormalities here, it is also as likely to imply what he might see as inappropriate relationships, and as he is specifying working-class women, many middle-class readers would accept this as normal for the vulgar lower orders who were not seen as having the moral backbone of the rest of society.

Culture, Art and Politics

In 1879 and 1899, fragments of copies on papyrus of the poems of Sappho, the ancient Greek female writer, were discovered in an astonishing way – some having been used as packing in burials of animals in Egypt and uncovered in archaeological digs. Sappho was born in the seventh century BCE on the Greek island of Lesbos and on her home island she gathered around her a circle of other female poets who became a form of same-sex community. Sappho wrote some beautiful poems to other women and it is thanks to her own expressions of her feelings for females, and the nature of her island community, that women in romantic relationships with each other have been referred to as 'lesbians'. At the time of the discovery little of her work survived, although she was known of and snippets had been passed on second hand, so these fragments were a revelation to academics and those educated and affluent enough to have the time to take it in. Consequently, in some circles and locations it became fashionable to be a 'Sapphist', as long as it remained a diversion and not an end in itself; the women involved, by and large, were expected to 'get it out of their system' and then settle

CHAPTER TWO

down with a husband (or be a Sapphist as some form of hobby whilst married). Paris was a notable example of a host for a Sapphist network, which developed in bohemian circles well before 1900 and continued after the First World War, when English author Radclyffe Hall was a regular patron of the lesbian haunts and social events – Hall even based some of the scenes and characters in her book *The Well of Loneliness* on people and venues she encountered there.

During the excitement caused by the discovery of the Sappho fragments, one man was still in deep mourning for the loss of his beloved and devoted companion and friend. In fact, in 1879 the survivor of the relationship – John Henry Newman (1801–1890) was made a Cardinal by Pope Leo XIII. This shy, scholarly man had met his closest companion, Ambrose St John (1815–1875) at about the time he helped found the Oxford Movement, which aimed to bring the Anglican Church back to its Catholic roots – at that time, Newman was a Church of England Deacon. Fourteen years Newman's junior, Ambrose was to become the closest person to Newman till the former's death. In 1845 both men were received into the Catholic Church and were ordained priests within their new spiritual home. The two men were together much of the time, and when Ambrose died, Newman threw himself on the bed in an agony of grief, staying with his dear friend all night; he continued to grieve till his own death, often reduced to tears at the very mention of Ambrose's name.

How to define this relationship between two loving, loved, shy priests? One must not attempt to put facts in, which – even if we are convinced they happened – we cannot prove. What we do know is this: Newman and Ambrose became devoted companions; they went through much adversity together when Newman had to resign as vicar of the university Church and his Oriel College fellowship, and caused a storm with his theologically challenging *Tract 90*; Newman wrote a heartfelt account of his friend in *Apologia Pro Vita Sua*, his account of his life and conversion to the Catholic faith. The two men did not lack courage, changing their faith, challenging existing ideas, and often severely censured for doing so. Newman was devastated when his companion died and, when it was his turn to meet his God, he was buried with his beloved in the graveyard by the home of the Oratory Fathers at Rednal Hill. Some people may ask: 'Yes, that's all very well, but were they lovers?' It is doubtful that researchers will ever know that. One could say that in their hearts, they loved each other deeply and consistently, for years, and parting was

53

agonizing when death came to one of them. In that sense surely, whether or not there were any sexual acts involved is irrelevant.

Sadly, not all loves between two men ended as gently as that of Ambrose and Cardinal Newman. The gifted artist Simeon Solomon (1840–1905) was arrested on 11 February 1873 along with one George Roberts and charged with committing an 'offence' at the public urinal in Stratford Place Mews, London. Although Solomon received a suspended sentence of eighteen months and only had to endure police supervision, his friends melted away and he eventually fell into penury and alcoholism. He ended up a wandering pavement artist and was arrested a second time for trying to steal gold leaf from the studio of Edward Burne-Jones, the famous artist; he died in St Giles Workhouse in 1905. Not even membership of an artistic elite could save a person from the shame and disgrace that condemnation of one's desires brought, as Oscar Wilde was famously to discover later in the century.

The Victorian era is widely regarded as the time when many of our great novels were written, but those written by women were often (at least initially) disguised as being by men, with a suitably masculine pen name. Charlotte Bronte published under the name of Currer Bell because it was felt that her work would be more readily received by the public that way. Gender was not the only thing that Charlotte was discreet about, however. In 1831, Charlotte met Ellen Nussey at school and their passionate friendship was to continue for many years till Charlotte's death in 1855. The hundreds of letters written by Charlotte to her love are testament to the strength of their bond, although Ellen's letters have not survived so we can only look at the relationship from one side; Charlotte had expressed a decision to destroy the letters sent to her by Ellen, and this may have been because of her marriage late in her life to Arthur Bell Nichols. He also wrote to Ellen demanding that she destroy the letters Charlotte wrote to her, as he objected to the passionate language in them – thankfully she scornfully rejected his request.

From the letters, we know that the two young women thought about setting up home together. In 1836, Charlotte wrote:

Ellen, I wish I could live with you always. I begin to cling to you more fondly than ever I did. If we had but a cottage and a competency [income] *of our own, I do think we might live and love on till Death without being dependent on any third person for happiness.*

CHAPTER TWO

These are strong sentiments for any person to write to another, and even leaving aside the fact that Charlotte liked to be independent financially and not have to rely on family, it seems clear that she preferred Ellen's company to anyone else's. It was never to be – Charlotte was only 20 years old at the time, and it was unlikely that her relatives would condone such a domestic arrangement, especially if they found out the depth of the feelings these young women had for each other. The only time it seemed likely was when Ellen's brother Henry proposed to Charlotte – she refused him, but did write that she was sorely tempted to say yes, simply in order to live under the same roof as Ellen. This relationship was no teenager's crush. It continued into adulthood, maturing into a relationship all too familiar to many with its expressions of affection and devotion, agonising separations, and rocky paths, at one point caused by the deep friendship Ellen developed with Amelia Ringrose in the 1840s. It seems that Charlotte was uncomfortable to the point of jealousy over this relationship, and the situation only eased when Amelia got married.

In 1853, Charlotte and Ellen had a bitter and damaging quarrel, possibly over Charlotte's decision to marry Arthur Bell Nichols, the curate at her father's church in Haworth. Having spent her whole life arguing against the married state, suddenly she was engaged, and Ellen was beside herself with jealousy and grief. The fact that Charlotte was doing this to provide security for her father in his old age was no compensation to anyone other than Charlotte; her only expression of happiness as a married woman was on this pragmatic level. Sadly and inevitably, Charlotte and Ellen could not go on as before. Nichols was determined to undermine the bond between them and often prevented them spending time together. After Charlotte died in 1855, author Elizabeth Gaskell was commissioned to write Charlotte's biography, and she even included in it some passionate notes between the two women. Clearly Mrs Gaskell thought it was acceptable in their day to have a passionate friendship between two women, even if the reality was that the husband in this case could not cope with the rivalry to his own dominance.

Edward Carpenter and the Campaign for Acceptance and Understanding

In 1882, the father of a man named Edward Carpenter (1844–1929) died, leaving his son an inheritance of £6,000 – the equivalent of approximately

£660,000 today. This sort of money would be enough to tempt anyone to live a champagne lifestyle, but for Carpenter, it meant the freedom to campaign for the causes he held dear. Having already resigned as an Anglican curate in the early 1870s, he had been making a living of sorts as a travelling lecturer in the North of England, and so it was in Millthorpe near Sheffield that he chose to buy a smallholding, took up market gardening and sandal making, and helped set up a local socialist group. He spoke in favour of nationalisation and in support of communal farms, and his cottage home became a venue for radicals and fellow socialists to meet and debate. Carpenter was also a man who loved the company of other men, having a similar approach to the ideal of the brotherhood of manly love as the American poet, Walt Whitman, and shied away from effeminate men and overly aesthetic mannerisms – his belief was that most men who had same-sex feelings were much more masculine than that, and to him, the latter were the 'perfect types', and the phrase 'dear love of comrades' or 'comradeship' was a coded way of talking about homosexual relationships without implying any effeminacy. Some years after he set up his smallholding he met George Merrill, who was to be his lifelong companion from that time till Merrill's death in 1928. They eventually settled at the Millthorpe cottage together, but whereas the local community had been sanguine about Carpenter's political beliefs, they were not nearly so accepting of his new male partner moving in and becoming the home maker for them both, a situation not helped by George's disingenuous openness about his homosexuality.

With this loving relationship to buoy him, in 1884 Carpenter joined the Fellowship of the New Life (the genesis of the Fabian Society) and here met sexologist Havelock Ellis, upon whom he had a profound influence. Carpenter was proud of his sexuality and his love for his partner, and when writing about what he called 'homogenic love', he was at pains to point out the many examples from history and in every society. He stated that a love like his was congenital (inborn and natural to that person), impossible to change and that it did not differ 'from the rest of mankind or womankind'. In doing so he also rejected the widespread idea of his times, and one that his former profession as a minister would have drummed into him: that a partnership between two people must have the primary aim of reproduction. In addition, as a committed socialist, Carpenter lectured at meetings of the Independent Labour Party and also to the Fellowship of the New Life, all the while working hard on his writings about sexuality;

by the end of the 1890s, his work *Homogenic Love and it's Place in a Free Society* was ready to be published. Sadly, thanks to the adverse publicity created by the Oscar Wilde trials, he could not find a publisher until a small print run for a private circulation was produced by the Manchester Labour Press. This he expanded and published again as *The Intermediate Sex* in 1908. The book slipped into the bookshops without a fuss, even making several reprints, and Carpenter went on in 1914 to found the British Society for the Study of Sex Psychology (BSSSP) with Lawrence Housman, which aimed to discuss matters around women's sexuality and homosexuality openly and honestly and which, as one of a number of aims, campaigned to have homosexuality decriminalised. Carpenter also found himself the recipient of many frank and touching letters from others of the 'intermediate sex' who had read his work and felt compelled to contact him. One woman, known only as KO, wrote to him of her terrible loneliness, even though his writings had confirmed for her who she was; she wrote of her longing to meet a female life partner, but also of the difficulties of meeting like-minded women. It could be said that Edward Carpenter and his works – and his open and honest love for his partner – were ground-breaking, and set a standard for others joining the campaign for equality to live up to, even if some of his ideas were a little too Utopian to be practical.

Another book, *A Problem in Greek Ethics*, was written by John Addington Symonds (1840–1894) and published in 1883, slightly before Carpenter started to write his own pleas for acceptance. It was a study of homosexuality in ancient Greece and the author, a respectable married man of middle-class background with a secret life of same-sex relationships (which he makes reference to in his memoirs), was a staunch campaigner for the repeal of Britain's sodomy laws. He later collaborated with Havelock Ellis on the book Sexual Inversion, published in 1897.

Sapphism and New Women in the Late Nineteenth Century

Culturally, the discovery of the Sappho poetry continued to have an impact. In 1877, two years before the find, Renee Vivien was born; she grew up to be a young woman of striking but ethereal beauty, and an avowed Sapphist and celebrator of love between women. She had the luxury of coming from a wealthy family and was able to indulge her literary interests. It would seem that her first passionate but platonic love was Violet Shileto, whom she met in Paris and continued to love throughout her life; but in 1899, she also developed a romance with writer Natalie Barney (1876–1972), who was so taken with Renee's beauty that she called her 'My angel'. Once again Renee saw her love as fine and pure, and wrote much poetry about it; seemingly she did not want to add any sexual element to it – yet was deeply upset when Natalie was not faithful to her. Her enduring love, Violet, died in 1901 and Renee never recovered from the grief; she was to die herself in 1909, a victim of an eating disorder and drug and alcohol dependency.

The education of women was improving all the time in the nineteenth century. The 1870 and 1880 Education Acts finally enabled all girls and boys to access a basic education no matter what their background and this was to lead to a new generation of people who had enough education to express their thoughts and feelings formally on an array of subjects. However, not even the most affluent, well born and best educated of women could escape the call of domestic responsibilities.

Frances Power Cobbe (1822–1904) came from an affluent Anglo–Irish, Protestant family and received an excellent education via tutors, schools and governesses. However, when Frances was 25, her mother died, and she had to take on the role of homemaker, looking after a large family of siblings and her father. This she did for eight years, and despite keeping up with her personal studies, always had the nagging feeling that her real life was in limbo. Following the death of her father in 1857, and armed with a small allowance from his will, Frances made her break for independence. After travelling abroad she began work in England as a pioneer in workhouse visiting, and collaborated with Mary Carpenter in her work with the Ragged and reformatory schools of Bristol. About two years later, Frances was introduced by a mutual friend to Mary Charlotte Lloyd, the woman who was to become the love of her life, her 'perfect friend', she was later to write, for 'thirty-four blessed years.' They eventually set up home together in Mary's house in London, and in the quarter of a century they were there, Frances established herself as a great campaigner on women's issues and for animal rights and welfare. She campaigned on behalf of women who had suffered domestic abuse, supported the suffrage movement which aimed to give women the vote, and believed that married women should be able to have their own property (this was achieved with the Married Women's Property Act of 1882). Eventually, as a mature couple Mary and Frances moved to North Wales, near Dolgellau, where they lived in Mary's family home of Hengwrt, a fairly remote, but stunningly beautiful part of the country, which was a welcome respite from the frantic pace of London and their campaigning. Mary died in 1896 and Frances in 1904, and they are buried together in a Llanelltyd graveyard near their historic home, with a fine headstone which faces the site of their beloved Hengwrt – there is a gentle irony in this as nearly all the other graves face in the opposite direction, to the East, and the same-sex lovers thus stand out in more ways than one in this tiny Welsh community.

The fact that Frances often described Mary as her 'friend' could be misleading as to the nature of their relationship. Many women who wished to describe their relationship discreetly referred to their partner or lover as a 'friend', and even today many female same-sex couples suffer the mild annoyance of having outsiders describe their spouse as their friend. Clearly, we cannot look beyond Frances and Mary's bedroom door and see how far that friendship went, and nor should we because all couples deserve privacy. An interest in the sex lives of historical figures can soon become gratuitous and distasteful if one ends up obsessively trying to build up a picture of a certain intimacy that cannot be proved or disproved. All we can say honestly is that these two women loved each other devotedly for many years, set up home together, supported and nursed each other probably better than many male–female couples did at that time. Perhaps they were the foremothers of the original 'lesbian-feminist' couples who were prevalent in the Women's Movement of the 1970s. Certainly their love was passionate, committed, and deep, as described in verses six and seven from a poem Frances wrote about Mary ('To Mary C Lloyd') in 1873:

Hereafter, when slow ebbs the tide,
And age drains out my strength and pride,
And dim-grown eyes and palsied hand
No longer list my soul's command,
I'll want you,– Mary.

In joy and grief, in good and ill,
Friend of my heart: I need you still,
My Guide, Companion, Playmate, Love,
To dwell with here, to clasp above,
I want you – Mary.

Another female pioneer was Sophia Jex-Blake (1840–1912), who was one of the first women in Britain to qualify and practice medicine in Britain. Born into a wealthy Sussex family and from an early age a forceful character, she always knew that it was to be women she would love, not men. Her first major love was Octavia Hill, whom she met at Queen's College in London. These two strong-minded women lived together for a year before Octavia's mother intervened, claiming that Blake was an adverse, overpowering influence on her daughter. Blake had to leave her lover, an event which deeply wounded her; she never forgot her first real love even though she had other female partners over the years, including Harriot Yorke, with whom she lived for the last thirty-five years of her life. The two women are buried together in the churchyard at Crockham Hill, near Edenbridge, in Kent.

In education, Constance Maynard (1849–1935) was a pioneer of higher education for women in Britain, and she was instrumental in the development of Westfield College in the University of London. She herself had been privileged to take advantage of the recently established Girton College in 1872, and it was during her three years there that she formed a passionate attachment to Louisa Lumsden, who referred to Constance as her 'wife'. The two young women moved to Scotland after graduating to further Louisa's teaching career, living together as any other married couple would. Sadly, religious differences forced them apart and Constance returned to London where her own career was to blossom, and she could pursue her devotion to her faith as she wished without Louisa's agnosticism getting in the way. She became the first head of Westfield College and remained so for over thirty years, but her faith did not stop her getting entangled in an emotional triangle with Anne Richardson and Frances Ralph Gray. Constance was a demanding element in the complex relationship and it forced 'Ralph' to move out of college for some peace, which Constance never forgave her for. This was just another romantic attachment that Constance made, there having been numerous 'crushes' in the past, even whilst living with Louisa.

One woman whose sexuality has been called into dispute is Lilian Baylis (1874–1937), and she is a good example of how historians have tried to put her into a particular category by using extrapolation based on her circle of acquaintance.

Lilian Baylis is probably best known for her involvement with two famous theatres, the Old Vic and Sadler's Wells, both of which she managed. She was the niece of Emma Cons, who actually founded the Old Vic, and Lilian herself performed in various ways in theatres both in Britain and abroad. Lilian lived for a long time with her aunt and another aunt, Ellen, until both her elders died, and so was well used to an all female environment. Historians know little about Lilian's domestic and private life other than this as she went to great lengths to 'cover her tracks', destroying most of her personal paperwork herself. Rosemary Auchmuty, who has researched the life of Lilian and her network of acquaintance, states: 'When women destroy all evidence of their personal lives, this should immediately alert us' (to the possibility that she may have had same-sex relationships). Auchmuty goes on to assert that it is possible to imply that Lilian was lesbian because of the identities of her close circle of friends. This circle included Winifred Holtby, the writer, and Ethel Smyth, the suffrage campaigner and composer; Ethel Smyth in turn knew many women who would now be 'pigeonholed' as lesbian or who had had same-sex relationships – Virginia Woolf, Edith Craig, Claire 'Tony' Atwood. Taking this circle a little wider, one can include Radclyffe Hall and her spouse Una. Why would a woman who preferred the company of men, spend nearly all her social life with women who, by and large, desired other women? Auchmuty states:

> [Baylis] *is interesting as an example of a woman whose circles of friends spread outwards from the local connections ... through the London theatrical and professional women's scene into a wider network of – what? Of unmarried, woman-centred women, many of whom were lesbians.*

Family historians may feel this is a dangerous game to play. Are we not simply doing what gossip mongers at the time would have done over the garden gate, assuming that someone is homosexual simply because some of their friends were? We are always told not to make assumptions or sweeping judgements in our genealogical research, yet sometimes an educated and well-researched judgement is necessary to move along one's research, so long as we are mindful that new evidence may come along and we must take it into account. It may be that Lilian preferred the company of assertive, independent, professional women because she was one herself, and had she mixed in more conventional social circles there may have been pressure on her, however subtle and covert, to marry and give over her life to a man. There is no evidence that Lilian had sexual relationships with other women, but she certainly enjoyed predominantly female company, which according to writer Adrienne Rich, constitutes a lesbian community of sorts. Perhaps as family historians we can take the idea of investigating a person's circle of acquaintances and do this for a person in our family's history who we think might have been homosexual, and see if such a same-sex 'network' emerges. It will then be up to the individual to judge on the evidence found what they think the conclusion should be.

By the late nineteenth century, working-class women who sought same-sex relationships were known as 'toms' or 'tommies', the term *tom* being familiar not only as a boy's name, but also used for male cats and masculine girls – 'tomboys'. However, it had previously been used as a term to describe sexually promiscuous women, even prostitutes, and as the century came to a close it was a term that put both categories of women into a transgressive minority group. Cat imagery, jokes and wordplay were also widely used to lampoon women in the suffrage movement, the idea of a 'catty woman' implying a sneaking nastiness and tendency to lash out at others, and a 'cat fight' meaning a fight between two women. Women in the suffrage movement were also depicted comically as either dried up old spinsters or overweight and overbearing harridans – women who were only drawn into this all female environment because, unlike 'real' women, they could not get themselves a man, and were therefore looking for female 'comfort '. Society was certainly consistent in its caricaturing of minority groups.

Case Study: The Masked Ball of 1880 in Manchester

Unfortunately, many of the people we have to study when researching same-sex relationships are people of education or 'good' family who actually came to public notice through their great works or community involvement, and it can be difficult to get a good balance of tales from all levels of society. However, the men who attended the masked ball on 25 September 1880 at the Temperance Hall in Hulme, Manchester, were very much of mixed backgrounds and came together for a common purpose – to meet like-minded people and enjoy themselves, as themselves, for just the one evening. It was a story that hit the headlines for a number of reasons.

The Temperance Hall was a drab looking building in a cul-de-sac accessed from York Street in Hulme, which could be hired for a variety of functions, and could accommodate in excess of 100 guests. At some point in the week before the incident, three men claiming to be from an organisation calling itself the Association of Pawnbroker's Assistants hired the room for the evening of 25 September. Two of the men were later arrested with other guests, but their names are not known. Later, it transpired that there had been a plan to hold several other events under the same booking, although these others never did take place. However, at some time before this particular event, a similar ball had taken place at a venue near Strangeways in Manchester, and there had possibly been others too, as the police had been on the lookout for such gatherings since the end of the previous year, which was why their suspicions were alerted when they heard about the false booking in Hulme. It later transpired that the association concerned knew nothing of the booking, and it seems that unknown persons had used their name as a cover to book for another covert group. Once the police had been alerted to the false booking, Detective Sergeant Caminada, a talented police officer who was making an name for himself as a tough and efficient policeman, was dispatched to the hall with a team of men to check out what was happening. They set about staking out the hall in good time, both in plain clothes and uniform, so that they were in place before any guests arrived. After 6.00pm, the man who dealt with the lettings for the hall met with two men there, later arrested, and opened up the place for them; Caminada later reported that the two men were in high spirits and laughing after the secretary had left. When people did start arriving at about 9.00pm, Caminada noted that the young men who alighted from the cabs had luggage of some kind with them, or they were dressed in 'female attire, and among the costumes were several low-bodied dresses.' (*Staffordshire Sentinel*, 2 October 1880). Forty-seven men were counted going into the building, twenty-two of whom were cross-dressed as women. Music from a harmonium was heard about an hour later, played by a blind man (presumably hired so he could not tell tales after the event!). At about 10.30pm, the police covertly watched as the secretary of the hall tried to gain entry to make sure all was above board. He was greeted by a man dressed as a Sister of Mercy, who insisted to the flustered secretary that they were just having a bit of fun and that the men dressed as women still had their 'proper' clothes on underneath (a statement he later repeated to the police). It was difficult for the police to see what was actually happening in the building because all the windows had been covered apart from two, which were open for ventilation. By climbing onto the roof of the hall's outhouse, Caminada could see into the hall via these windows, and from his observation post he watched events at the party unfold. He apparently saw that 'The company were engaged chiefly in grotesque dances, such as are familiar at lower-class music halls .... They danced some strange kind of dance, in which they kicked their legs about a great deal.' This referred to the can-can. The *Manchester Courier* breathlessly reported that of those in fancy dress or female attire:

> *the characters of historical and other personages* [were] *assumed .... "Juliet" was conspicuous among the grotesque assumptions. Bracelets and jewellery of a tawdry description were worn .... Among the personages represented by those in male attire were Romeo, Henry VIII, Richard III, Sir Walter Raleigh, and the Earl of Leicester.*

The cross-dressing men were largely dancing with men who were in male clothes, with even those seated around the sides of the room paired off into couples in this way. Another newspaper, the *Blackburn Standard*, reported the evidence of Caminada verbatim on 2 October: 'We could hear persons "squealing" and talking loudly in feminine voices, which they all affected.' At the same time, 'certain proceedings' were going on in an anteroom. Two other officers nearly gave the game away, when some debris fell from the roof on which they were standing; a guest came to investigate, but did not spot the police hiding there. It must have been an entertaining sight, as Caminada did not make a move until 1.00–2.00 pm in the morning! By this time he was satisfied of the 'impropriety' of events in the hall and after obtaining corroboration of his opinion from some plain-clothes police officers, he prepared his men for a raid. Quietly his team lined up against the building, ready for the signal to go in. Caminada knocked several times on the door, and eventually someone asked: 'Who's there?' From listening to the arrivals earlier Caminada knew that the password was 'Sister', which he then said whilst 'imitating a female voice'. As soon as the door opened, the police rushed in to the hall. 'A scene almost indescribable followed,' thundered the *Manchester Courier* on the following Monday, 27 September. Startled and afraid, some of the revellers lashed out, lunged at the police and tried to force them back onto the street; Caminada was thumped and thrown into the doorway. Caminada later told the court that: 'A free fight took place between the police and those in the room.' Unfazed, he grabbed hold of the two guests nearest to him and, with this signal, all those who could be apprehended by his colleagues, were. In the pandemonium, some guests tried to pull off their female clothes and were still trying when grabbed by officers; one man tried to escape into the street via a window, but gave up when he saw another sergeant waiting for him below. As many guests as possible were handcuffed, to prevent any further violence. One of the guests insisted that the cross-dressing guests were wearing their male clothes underneath their gowns, which proved not to be the case. Caminada presumably felt short handed bearing in mind the number of guests he had to deal with, as some men and a few women were called in from the street to help. Only one guest managed to make his escape, and was apprehended soon after, still wearing some of his female clothes. All the guests were handcuffed and eventually ended up at the cells in the Town Hall, which also housed the detective department. Large amounts of clothes were seized and taken away from the hall as evidence; pieces of costume jewellery were picked up off the pavement and road outside, where they had been thrown off or dropped in the confusion.

The following morning, no doubt after a night of distress, discomfort, and agonising worry about what family, friends and colleagues would say, the men were brought before the Manchester Police Court, still wearing the clothes in which they had been arrested. Word of the colourful events had spread quickly and curious spectators arrived in their droves at the court in the hopes of getting a seat to watch the spectacle, but the police sensibly kept the numbers admitted to a minimum. There were so many defendants that they could not all fit into the dock, and some had to sit on the benches usually reserved for members of the legal profession. Caminada led the giving of the evidence, stating what he observed and adding that he knew some of the men and that they were of 'bad character':

> *There exists a class of men, unknown to many gentlemen, who prowl about the streets almost to the same extent as unfortunate women, and some of the prisoners belong to that class.*

He was of course referring to his observation that some of the attendees were male prostitutes. Some of the men were visibly distressed and covered their faces to avoid the gaze of the members of the public in the gallery. The legal wrangling now began. Caminada asked for more time to prepare his case, as it had been decided to go ahead with a prosecution and requested that the arrested men should be remanded till Thursday with bail allowed as two sureties of £10 each if necessary. One solicitor, acting on behalf of two of the men, told the court that his clients had been misled as to the nature of the ball, and were businessmen of good standing who would find it a great difficulty to be in custody till Monday when bail was to be arranged; could it not be done that very day? Mr Rickards JP, presiding, retorted that after what he had heard that morning he had 'no sympathy for them at all', was 'not going to do them any favours whatsoever' and ordered that they all go back to the cells. Not all the men took their barracking meekly, however; 36-year-old George Bingham of Sheffield tried to explain why he should not be remanded:

> I do not see why I should be charged at all. I was asked if I would come to a fancy dress ball. I replied, "Well I don't know; I'll see. I went late last night, and as regards what the officer said about misconduct, I did not see much of it. I was in the room sat down. I did not dance once.

The magistrate replied sharply that because he had been present and 'very disgusting practices were being carried on', he was equally liable.

The following Thursday, all forty-seven men returned to the court, even though thirty-seven of them had been bailed; as they filed into the court they were jeered at by the gallery, with loud comments made about their appearance. They were now all in male clothes, however:

> Some of them were of gentlemanly appearance and demeanour, others were very effeminate in appearance, and the hair was presumably dyed the golden hue so much effected in quasi-fashionable circles. Their stations in life were evidently very different, some being well dressed, while others were not only shabby and unkempt, but evidently belonged to the lower classes of society.

The men were to be charged with a misdemeanour under common law, on the grounds that all of the men had incited each other to immorality, and a further charge was brought for conspiring together to assemble at a particular place and there to solicit and incite each other to commit improper actions. This was of course before the Labouchere Amendment of 1895, so a charge of gross indecency was still fifteen years into the future. The men in the dock must have been terrified to hear that it was an offence that could land them in prison for up to ten years. Thankfully, the magistrates were not minded to clutter up the prisons with these men, and they decided that rather than a custodial sentence, each one was to 'enter into their own recognisances in the sum of £50, and find two sureties of £25 each, to be of good behaviour for twelve months, the alternative being three months imprisonment.' Until the sureties could be arranged, the men were to remain in custody.

By 2 October the *Derby Telegraph* was recording the amazement of locals at how leniently the forty-seven men had been treated, although it was also revealed that the poorer men, who were mostly local to Manchester and Salford, could not raise the £25 sureties and would have to serve three months in gaol if it could not be found – no wonder when, in modern money, there would not be much change from £5,000, certainly an impossible sum for any of the labourers to raise, unless they had affluent friends amongst their circle of same-sex acquaintance.

This is a fascinating case, reported in detail certainly in the local and provincial newspapers, because of its unusual storyline and also perhaps because Caminada was a rising star of the local police force, and the press followed his career with interest. So far we know what happened, and we know that there were forty-seven men involved. But who were they? Historians are extremely fortunate that the press took such glee in reporting this case, because along with other sources one can make a list of the men, their personal details, and in some cases, track them through records such as the census to see how and where they lived, and what their family was like. A complete list of the men is given in Appendix Two, but some examples follow of the attendees of the ball who have so far been found in the records. Before we make the acquaintance of some of these men, in summary it can be said that the age range was 16 to 48 years, approximately thirty of them were single, and the rest have unknown marital status or were married. They all claim to have work of some kind – presumably only those in work could afford to have the money to attend the party and buy, make, or hire clothes for it – and the range of jobs indicates a spectrum of social levels. Many were from the Manchester area, but approximately a quarter were from Sheffield, and a few other places were represented by individuals, such as Stockport, Stalybridge and Ashton -under- Lyne.

Any researcher following this case has the advantage of the 1881 census, which happened only months later, and thankfully some of the men can readily be found. In 1881, James Lythgoe was living with his family at 13, Wallman Road, Salford; his father Cornelius, who was in his sixties, was a tailor. Interestingly, James was born in Hulme so it is possible that he spent some of his childhood there and knew the area to a degree. He does not have any occupation listed on the census, so it is likely that he lost his job as a clerk after the court case. The address is also different but people moved around so much at that time because, as tenants, it was easy to do, so it is impossible to say if the move was connected to any backlash from neighbours at the old address in Salford. In 1891 the family had moved again, to Doddington Street; James was still living at home with his parents and was listed as a clerk once again.

Henry Parry was still working as a painter in 1881, and still living at the same address of 6, Fern Court in Hulme; perhaps, as a local lad, his neighbours knew him and were more likely to accept him for who he was. He was lodging with a widow and her adult daughter, and it looks like a poor household; the mother was a waste picker, and her 20-year-old daughter was a matchbox maker, a piece-work activity normally done at home and very badly paid.

Abraham Ogden is still listed as a baker, but has moved to another address in Hulme – 5, Duke Street – where he was living with a large extended family of nine , the householder being his Uncle, an upholsterer; also living there is his 72-year-old mother. Arthur Shawcross, who had been born in Stalybridge, was still working too, as a mechanic, and had moved from West Gorton to Openshaw (an adjacent district) where he was living alone at 12, Bell Street. By 1891 he had moved to Blackpool, and was living on his own means (either savings or some form of pension or insurance payment) and was sharing 5, Thomas Street with one John W. Dunkerley, a Mancunian in his twenties who was working as a general clerk. Are Arthur and John partners, and did they move to Blackpool so they could live their lives quietly and in anonymity, away from the gossips who knew them too well? We cannot know for sure that they are in a relationship, but one hopes for a happy and settled ending for Arthur, by now in his late fifties.

George Buxton surfaces on the 1901 census, at 3, Robinson Court, Ardwick, where he was boarding with 28-year-old John Jones, who is the head of the household. John is a fish hawker, more than likely someone who carried his wares around the streets selling them; George was still a fustian cutter (a hand finishing process in textile manufacture). Walter Smith, a 22-year-old fruit hawker from the Midlands, was also staying there and listed as a visitor. All three men are listed as single. With Walter being listed as a visitor, the household is officially just John and George. Again, are they a couple? We have no way of knowing just from this census entry.

Alfred Buckmaster has a slightly more upmarket household; he had not moved far after the court case and was still at Albion Place, Cheetham, albeit a few doors from his old address. He lived with his sister Mary, who was listed as the housekeeper, and they had two rather impressive boarders – 26-year-old John Lewis, a professor of music, and Edward Mellor, a mathematics teacher. Alfred has described himself as a shipping agent. Ten years previously, in 1871, Alfred Buckmaster was a 17-year-old clerk still living at home in his native Liverpool with his family; his father Henry was Registrar of births, marriages and deaths. More questions arise. Did Alfred leave Liverpool because of his sexuality, and settle in Manchester to enjoy the freedom of his own actions away from any fear of bringing shame on his relatives? Was he forced to do so? It would not be unusual for someone in his position to flee the family fold in order to live and love according to his needs and wishes.

Originally a waiter, by 1881 Nathaniel Saxton had changed address from Grove Street in Sheffield and was lodging with a married couple, their 3-year-old child, and another boarder at 72, Tagus Street in that city. He is listed as what appears to be a publican's waiter, possibly a 'potman' collecting up the glasses and so on. Ten years later Nathaniel's life had changed considerably. He had married Ellen Jane Robinson in Sheffield in 1890, and they were living at 2 Court, 6, Infirmary Road; Nathaniel is a carter. Move forward another ten years to 1901 and the couple have moved to 352, Cricket Street; they have no children listed, but shared their home with an adult nephew and niece. Nathaniel was a railway porter. He died in 1924. One should be careful not to immediately read a story into the childlessness of Nathaniel and Ellen, because at this time infant mortality was such that they might have had children who had died between census returns and at that time, still births would not be recorded; tempting though it would be to suggest that this was a marriage of convenience to cover for Nathaniel's homosexuality, one cannot do that. The idea that someone who seeks partners of the same sex cannot also dearly love a person of the opposite gender at all is untenable. He may have loved Ellen all the more if she knew exactly who he was, and covered for and protected him; at a time of restrictive moral attitudes, that would have been a selfless and indeed courageous thing for her to do.

Ernest John Parkinson lived with his large family at Victoria House, Frederick Street, Bury, as he had done at the time of his arrest; on the census he is described as a comedian rather than a singer. His father is a brassfounder employing twenty-one people, so Ernest probably had some protection from the fact that his family was affluent and therefore had status locally. In 1911, Ernest was living in Hulme, still with some family, and working as a musician. His two brothers, Samuel and Arthur, whom he lived with, were also single like him. One wonders what memories of that stressful evening decades before came flooding back to Ernest when he moved to the area where the masked ball was held. It was noted by newspapers at the time of the ball that Ernest worked with Tute's Minstrels, and it is thought that he was a female impersonator – perhaps on the night of the masked ball, he even performed for what would have been an appreciative audience.

Charles Speed was still at his given address in Monmouth Street, Sheffield, in 1881, and engaged in the same work as a silver finisher; he has a 30-year-old boarder named Henry Kirkby, and a visitor is listed – a German man aged 33, Louis Schultz, who worked as a butler. Once again, can we guess that Charles and Henry are partners? Charles, as head of household, certainly could not put down 'husband' for Henry on the census form, even if that is how he regarded him; the days of marriage equality were over a century away. It would be sensible for him to put boarder instead, which suggests a long term lodger but is completely respectable in a working-class area where most households helped pay their way by taking in paying guests.

Two other men are worthy of note, because they both gave the same address when arrested: George Broughton, a school master aged 30, and 25-year-old draper John Cartwright, both of 62, Wakefield Road, Stalybridge. John was cross-dressing on the night of the ball. It is reasonable to think that George and John, as they lived together, also travelled to the event together, and they make the strongest case for being romantic partners out of all the men who can be traced. Sadly, neither man can be identified for sure in all the census returns – their relatively common names do not make them stand out even if they subsequently went their separate ways and married, moved away or found other partners. They may even have changed their names, as with the other men who are hard to track down. In addition, George's occupation as a teacher must have been in great peril; the school term would have been well under way when he was arrested and his absence would have been hard to explain away. The chances of his keeping his job would have been limited.

One person who has proved impossible to find is Frederick Montrasser. He claimed to be a waiter at Farbon's restaurant in Manchester, but he is nowhere to be seen in any census, even if one is very generous with spelling variations of his surname. The obvious conclusion is that he used an alias when arrested, perhaps even using a false name whilst working as a waiter, and until the mystery of his true identity is solved – if ever – one cannot hope to find out how he fared upon his release.

What does this case, reported with glee and in great detail by the press in the North West and elsewhere, tell us about men at the time who wished to socialise with each other? We are told in the reports that the men all knew each other, and were part of a network or 'private society' of acquaintance that met regularly to hold similar events; the *Manchester Courier* said teasingly: 'The correspondence which passes between them relative to different engagements is, we are informed, of an extraordinary description' but so far as researchers are aware, none of this has survived. What it does tell us, however, is that men from across diverse areas, occupations and social classes were willing to socialise on a regular basis at a variety of venues (no doubt changed for security purposes) in order to relax with people who would not judge them, but instead had an innate understanding of each other. It is little surprise that some of the names and addresses are hard to trace; to take on an alias and a false address, even in the face of police questioning, must have felt like the only way out of a terrifying situation. All these men claimed to have work, and no doubt some were in danger of losing that work had this scandal reached their employers; however, of those who can be located in records afterwards, most seem to have hung on to their jobs, but whether that was with the same employer, it is impossible to say. Certainly these men must have had a sense of community within their social group, and if there were block bookings of such events as was suggested in the reports, they would have made friends and even found lovers amongst their group. For some it must have been exciting to take the risk of discovery – the Temperance Hall was in a closely built district of mainly small terraced houses, and their comings and goings must have been observed by casual passers-by. For others the events must have been a lifeline, the only way they could meet and socialise with men who felt as they did; for yet others, it must have felt like the most natural thing in the world.

Regarding the cross-dressing, as the ball was fancy dress it was possible to claim that dressing as a woman was all part of the charade, but for others it may well have been a truer representation of their real feelings about their 'gender identity' as one might put it today. Like so many other aspects of events such as this, these are questions we cannot answer with any real integrity. What we can surmise is that these were not the only events of their kind in the nation, and that others went ahead unhindered time and again. Where people feel a real need to gather together, throughout history they have found a way, bound together by adversity and camaraderie. Looking back at the events and venues previously described in this narrative, there is a clear pattern emerging. Private societies or clubs were by far the safest way for men in particular to meet and socialise, as they would be known to each other and there was less chance of the police or any other unfriendly agents infiltrating the group. This was a pattern that continued well into the second half of the twentieth century, when lesbian and gay clubs were private clubs, and one was 'vetted' and questioned through a peep hole in the door before being allowed in. The progress towards completely open venues where one can mix with ease with other homosexuals has been slow and sometimes faltering.

The Cleveland Street Scandal

Cleveland Street, London, was a fairly typical street in the nation's capital in 1889. The terraced houses looked respectable and anonymous, which suited Charles Hammond, the proprietor of number 19, perfectly. Hammond ran a male brothel at this address, which only seemed to come alive at night as carriages dropped off affluent male clients on a regular basis. In July of that year, some money went missing from the premises of the Central Telegraph Office where 15-year-old Thomas Swinscow worked. Thomas was accused of stealing the money when he was found to have fourteen shillings in his pocket, but he vigorously denied this, claiming that he had earned the money at his evening employment. When pressed for details, he confessed that he worked as a male prostitute at Hammond's premises.

A police raid was conducted at number 19 and the working boys taken into custody, but Hammond was nowhere to be seen. In his absence, police began to question the boys to obtain the names of clients. By and large they did not know their names, but one was identified – the son of

CHAPTER TWO

the Duke of Beaufort, one Sir Arthur Somerset. Somerset moved in the highest circles, including the social set of the Prince of Wales.

Far from being castigated in the newspapers, the young male prostitutes were treated sympathetically by the press, who claimed they were victims of a dissolute and exploitative upper class. Clearly action had to be taken to satisfy public opinion, and a warrant for the arrest of Somerset was issued on the gross indecency with other males. He fled to the continent, where he remained till he died in 1926; Hammond also fled, to Canada, and never did have to account for his business activities. As was usually the case, the gap in the 'market' left by the collapse of his establishment would soon have been filled by another enterprising business person.

Oscar Wilde, the Trials and his Legacy

And all men kill the thing they love,
By all let this be heard,
Some do it with a bitter look,
Some with a flattering word,
The coward does it with a kiss,
The brave man with a sword!

(Verse from *The Ballad of Reading Gaol*, 1897; based on
Wilde's experiences as a convict)

In late Victorian England and beyond, Oscar Wilde was a feted celebrity, writer and raconteur. Born in Ireland in 1854, Wilde was a gifted and amusing writer with an easy charm but a rather foolish belief that these attributes would enable him to outrun the legal system. Wilde was a hugely popular playwright with hits such as *The Importance of Being Earnest* (1895) and had gathered around him a coterie of admiring aesthetes and handsome young men. Like many people who were drawn to romances with their own gender at that time, he was respectably married, to Constance (formerly Lloyd), and had two sons whom he apparently adored. He was fond of his wife and appreciated her quiet charm and reserve, but by the 1890s he had tired of married life and had returned to his close friendships with men. The fact that Wilde had extra-marital relationships was nothing of note amongst men of his standing at that time, in fact it was almost expected and thus, in a way, condoned;

73

however, Wilde's obvious chosen partners were men younger than himself, and for the most part rather beautiful to look at. The stunningly good looking John Gray (1866–1934) met Wilde in 1889 and they had a short relationship; there is also a striking resemblance between Gray and the character Dorian Gray in *The Picture of Dorian Gray*, which Wilde wrote in the year they met. The 'real' Gray's languid manner and blonde good looks were exactly the sort of ideal of beauty that Wilde appreciated, not just as a homosexual but as an aesthete and man of culture. It was his misfortune that he felt most strongly for another attractive blonde, Lord Alfred 'Bosie' Douglas, whose father was the volatile Marquess of Queensberry. When Queensberry found out that his son was associating with Wilde, he flew into a rage and, against the advice of friends, left a note at the Albermarle, Wilde's gentleman's club, accusing him of being a 'somdomite' [sic]. Wilde was humiliated and furious, and again, against the advice of friends, took Queensberry to court for libelling him in April 1895. Not brave enough to implicate his own son in the case, Queensberry hired investigators to identify working-class male partners that Wilde had associated with, a ploy that worked as Douglas never appeared in court as a witness. Although most of Wilde's work could not be taken as overtly homoerotic, his only novel, *The Picture of Dorian Gray* (1890) was strongly criticised in court for its 'dubious' subject matter. Consciously or otherwise, Oscar decided to treat the courtroom as some form of theatrical event – some commentators have suggested that Wilde's laissez-faire manner, his ready quips and his witty 'one liners' were a grave error of judgement and that he might have done better to present himself as a sober yet artistic man of standing.

Wilde stepped out of court defeated, but worse was to come; he was arrested under the Criminal Law Amendment Act on a charge of gross indecency, and he was subjected to another humiliating trial.

The legal proceedings and court hearings ground on, with Wilde suffering greatly in prison on remand (the magistrate, Sir John Bridge, could have granted bail but considered sodomy to be so vile that any alleged perpetrator did not deserve it). On 24 April, in order to pay Queensberry's £600 costs, Wilde's effects went into a bankruptcy sale – even his books and manuscripts. Two days later the trial began. After a month in captivity Wilde was anxious and looked unwell and careworn, thinner than before and with his hair much shorter, but he tried hard to maintain his elegance of phrase and his composure. One answer he gave

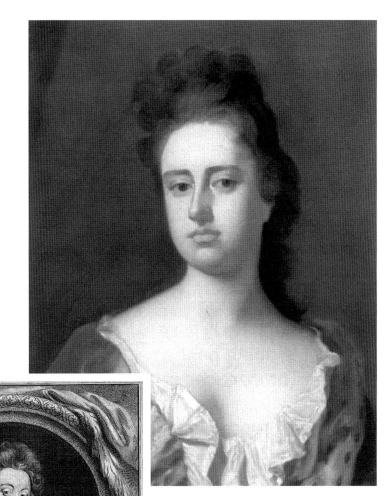

Queen Anne (above) and the woman she loved for years, Sarah, Duchess of Marlborough – a passionate and devoted friendship that sadly ended in acrimony.

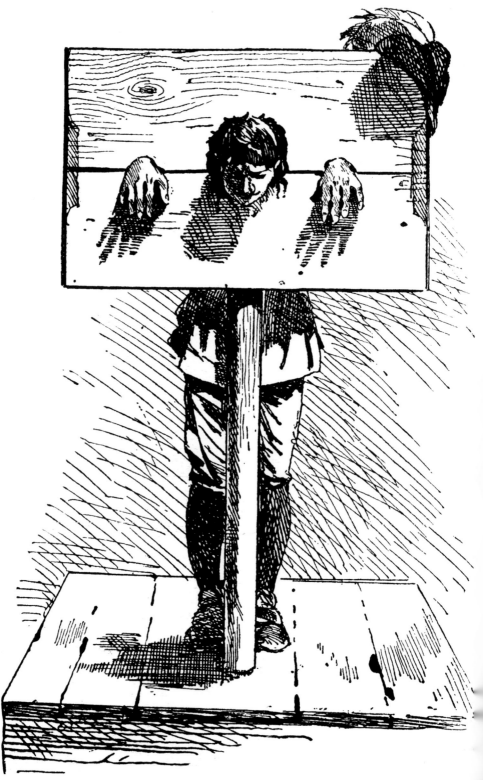

The Pillory, a commonly used method of punishing and humiliating sodomists. The miscreants were pelted with every kind of missile, including stones, dung, vegetables and dead animals.

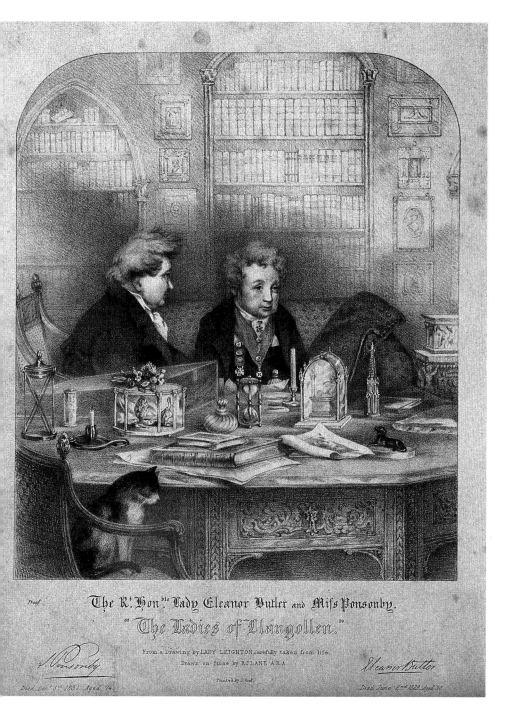

The Rt. Honble. Lady Eleanor Butler and Mifs Ponsonby.

"The Ladies of Llangollen."

From a Drawing by LADY LEIGHTON, carefully taken from life.
Drawn on Stone by R.J.LANE A.R.A.

Printed by J. Graf.

Ponsonby

Eleanor Butler

Died Dec.r 8th 1831. Aged 74.

Died June 2nd 1829. Aged 90.

e "Ladies of Llangollen", who set up home together at Plas Newydd, Llangollen, North Wales,
1780 and remained there together till Eleanor died in 1829.

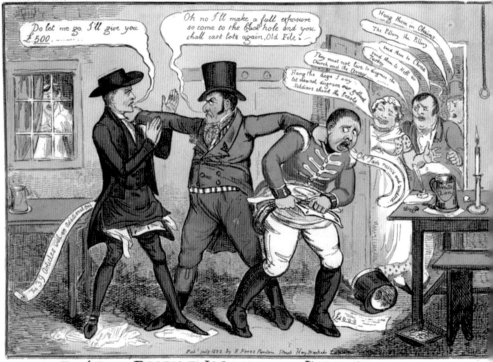

One of many satirical drawings of the scandal which led to the downfall of Percy Jocelyn, the Anglican Bishop of Clogher, who in 1822 was caught literally with his trousers down in the company of John Moverley, a Grenadier Guardsman.

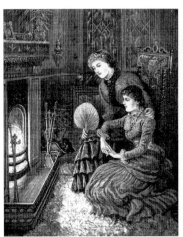

Intense, even passionate friendships or bonds between women – even if married – were an accepted expression of same-sex affection until the advent of the first wave feminist movement in the late nineteenth century.

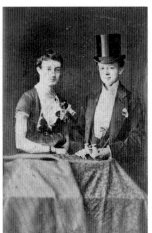

A late Victorian cabinet photograph, depicting a young woman in male attire on the right. As nothing is known about the woman, one cannot assume anything about her sexuality or gender identity simply because of her clothes.

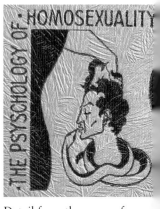

Detail from the cover of *Strange Lust: The Psychology of Homosexuality* by A M L Hesnard, one of many texts exploring the newly medicalis 'condition' of homosexuality

THE ILLUSTRATED POLICE NEWS

LAW-COURTS AND WEEKLY RECORD

DISGRACEFUL PROCEEDINGS IN MANCHESTER—MEN DRESSED AS WOMEN

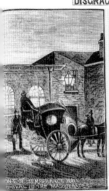

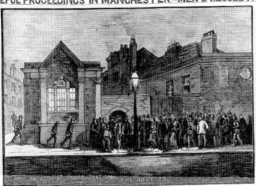

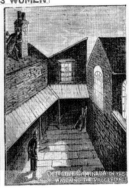

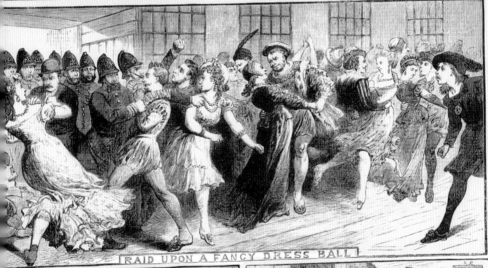

RAID UPON A FANCY DRESS BALL

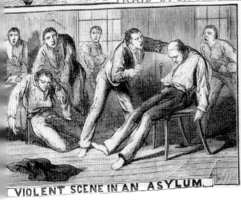

VIOLENT SCENE IN AN ASYLUM

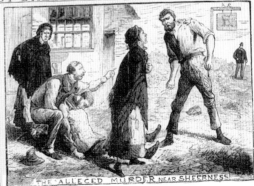

THE 'ALLEGED' MURDER NEAR SHEERNESS

masked ball in Hulme, Manchester, 1882. The dramatic scenes at the event were perfect for sensation-seeking readers of the *Illustrated Police News*.

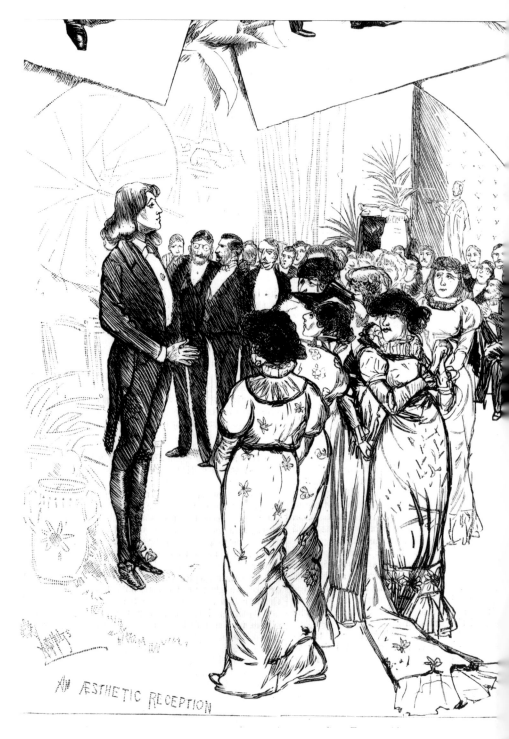

AN ÆSTHETIC RECEPTION

Oscar Wilde (left) entertaining fellow aesthetes with his famous wit on his American tour, 1882

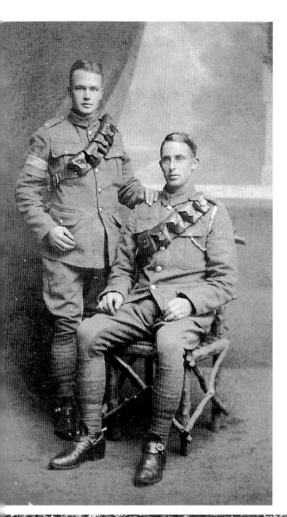

Two First World War soldiers. The deep, often loving, friendships forged in wartime were vital to the psychological well-being of many servicemen and women.

A group of British nurses, early twentieth century. Nursing was one of the professions that allowed women to be economically independent – and had the added advantage of offering inclusion in an all female community.

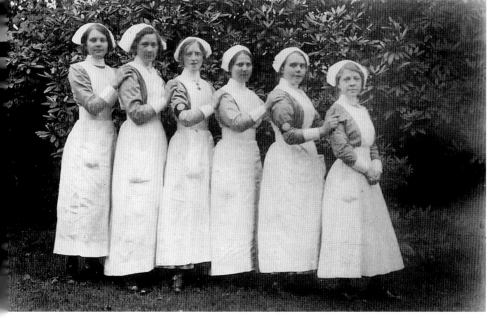

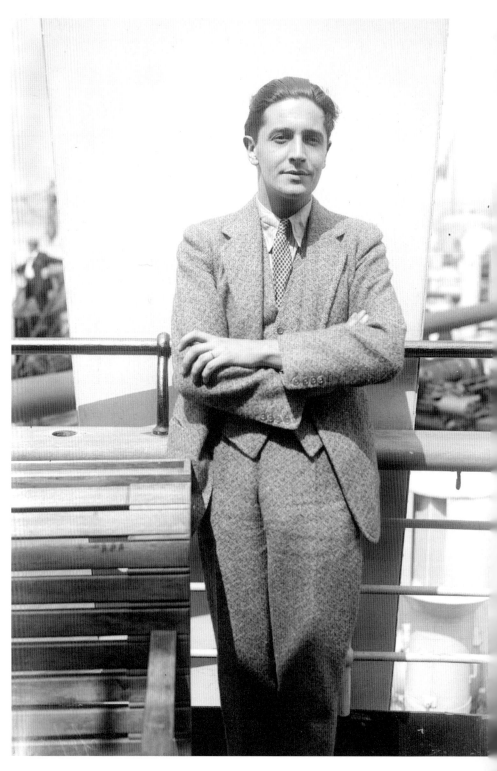

Ivor Novello, the hugely popular entertainer whose long term relationship with his partner Bob was concealed from the public – most other homosexual public figures were equally secretive.

in response to vigorous questioning about issues of sexuality has survived as a beautiful and succinct summary of how Wilde felt about same-sex attraction. In answer to cross examination by Mr C. F. Gill, who asked 'What is "the love that dare not speak its name" (a reference to a line in a poem)?' Wilde said:

> *"The Love that dare not speak its name" in this century is such a great affection of an elder for a younger man as there was between David and Jonathan, such as Plato made the very basis of his philosophy, and such as you find in the sonnets of Michelangelo and Shakespeare. It is that deep, spiritual affection that is as pure as it is perfect. It dictates and pervades great works of art like those of Shakespeare and Michelangelo, and those two letters of mine, such as they are. It is in this century misunderstood, so much misunderstood that it may be described as the "Love that dare not speak its name," and on account of it I am placed where I am now. It is beautiful, it is fine, it is the noblest form of affection. There is nothing unnatural about it. It is intellectual, and it repeatedly exists between an elder and a younger man, when the elder man has intellect, and the younger man has all the joy, hope and glamour of life before him. That it should be so the world does not understand. The world mocks at it and sometimes puts one in the pillory for it.*

Wilde, master of the poetic, was applauded for this statement, although there were a few who hissed him too, and the prosecutor, Edward Carson, was not impressed by his beautiful words, scorning Wilde's involvement with the working-class boys he 'picked up' as evidence of the gutter behaviour of an effeminate poseur. This trial ended with a hung jury and so Wilde had to endure yet another beginning on 22 May; three days later he was finally convicted. Coincidentally, it was Queen Victoria's birthday, and both the spectators at the court and subsequently the press, lambasted Wilde and his co-defendant, Alfred Taylor, for their unpatriotic activities.

There is little doubt that Wilde was made an example of, although his sentence was not out of the ordinary – the maximum sentence of two years hard labour, during which Wilde had to endure oakum picking (the pulling apart of short lengths of rope in order to recycle it) – but he became so ill that he was put on lighter duties instead. He left prison in 1897 a physically broken and spiritually defeated man, abandoned

Britain and ended the last few years of his life abroad, dying in Paris in 1900. An attempted reconciliation with Bosie did not work although they did spend some time together; Oscar was hurt and wretched, and felt that Bosie had not stood by him when it mattered. Henry Labouchere, who had put forward the amendment that essentially brought about Oscar's downfall, wrote of his disappointment that Wilde had received so short a sentence – Labouchere had originally proposed a maximum seven-year sentence in his amendment but this was rejected by parliament.

The impact of these trials on Wilde, his associates and his family was crushing. His wife Constance divorced him and he was never to see his beloved children again, despite his being a doting and delightful father. Most of Wilde's friends either deserted him in an emotional sense, or fled the country for fear of getting caught up in a follow-up persecution of his circle of acquaintance. Some friends remained loyal; one did not run away and in fact he visited Wilde in prison – More Adey. To the furious disappointment of Constance, Wilde welcomed these visits from his eccentric but devoted friend. Constance wrote to her husband: 'I require you to assure me that you will never see him again, or any of that kind.' Nevertheless, on 19 May 1897, it was Adey who was waiting for Oscar at the gates of Reading Gaol on his release. Robert 'Robbie' Ross, another of Wilde's loyal and devoted friends, also visited Wilde in prison, reciting to Oscar the poems from A. E. Housman's poetry collection *A Shropshire Lad*, which were partly inspired by the trial and imprisonment of Wilde as well as other influences that had affected the homosexual poet. When Oscar was released from prison, Housman sent him a copy of the book.

The trial was big news, and came at a time when more and more working-class and poor people had some literacy skills so could appreciate what headlines and news stories were telling them; newspapers, both national and provincial, were avidly read and the stories discussed over a many a garden gate and in pubs and clubs everywhere. Men in particular who sought out same-gender partners must have felt a mixture of fear, apprehension and possibly even self-dislike as their feelings for other men were torn apart in Wilde's trials. By proxy, they too were branded as perverts and the lowest of the low, and for some, to see in print how the legal system and society regarded them must have been a shock; the trials of Oscar Wilde were, of course, repeated across the country many times over, with less important or affluent players in the drama, but the effects would have been life changing whatever the status of the men involved.

CHAPTER TWO

The cultural implications of Oscar Wilde as a person, unwittingly standing in a courtroom as a spokesman for other men who fell in love with men, were also far reaching. Before Oscar's trials, an effeminate man was simply that – one not achieving the Victorian ideal of manliness, but not necessarily a man who had leanings towards relationships with other men. Charles Kingsley had stated in 1853 that he thought he lived in an effeminate age, and had described the Romantic poet Percy Bysshe Shelley as 'shrieking, railing, hysterical, tender, pitiful', but that does not necessarily mean he was accusing Shelley of being a sodomite. Hysterical is an apt choice of word if one was describing the effeminacy of a man, as it refers of course to high emotional states caused by a woman's hormones and uterus, but it does not necessarily mean that he is attracted to other men sexually. Wilde had long been flamboyant – from 1877 he had consciously adopted the appearance of an effeminate aesthete, and from 1882 he was more of an effeminate dandy, going from 'artistic' clothes to more flamboyantly tailored, even theatrical outfits, but if there were rumours about him, they were not associated with his appearance too closely. Indeed, if some historians are to be believed, until 1877 Wilde had had no same-sex intimacies, and would not until he had a relationship with Robert Ross in 1886. Nobody seemed to mind that poets and artists were effeminate, as that could be expected of the artistic temperament in the years of Wilde's youth. Alan Sinfield has suggested that the effeminate appearance and behaviours of Wilde were what led to a confusion between an 'artistic' or effete presentation, and a man who was attracted to other men, which in turn was to lead to many a limp-wristed comic character in movies and later in television programmes right into the second half of the twentieth century. His appearance and behaviour, it has been said, has subliminally suggested to generations of homosexual men that they had to model their own behaviour on him and be camp too. Wilde would have been horrified. He saw himself as having noble, self-sacrificing feelings for his lovers, feelings of romance that rivalled the great Greek loves themselves. For him, the 'love that dare not speak its name' was not unspeakable because it was vulgar, animalistic and crude; it was not to be articulated because it was so beautiful, it could not be spoken of by mere mortals. Faced with evidence of his supposed cultural legacy, he would more than likely have made some amusing quip, left the room and gone back to his artistic endeavours and high romances.

Oscar Wilde may have been deluding himself, but he does illustrate an aesthetic 'last stand' against the populist notion that all same-sex attraction was low and crude, and it was his trial that may well have accelerated the media attacks on men who were not fine examples of British manliness. Wilde was seen as a sham, a man who professed artistic sensibilities but beneath the veneer, was no better than a ghastly and perverted guttersnipe who had the audacity to push the issue of male same-sex desire into the public arena and onto the front pages of many a newspaper in middle-class parlours across the country. It is easier for a detractor to see someone else's actions or preferences as unpleasant and unhealthy because it quickly gives one the moral high ground, and this is what Wilde fought against, even within himself. He had to see beauty in his sexuality and his aestheticism, and in what he did, to think well of himself and his feelings. His opponents had to see him as dirty and a sexual predator in order to justify their treatment of him and others like him. His very name became a term of insult – to be homosexual was to 'be' Oscar Wilde, unclean and deserving of punishment and public scorn. A character in E. M. Forster's novel *Maurice* stated: 'I'm an unspeakable of the Oscar Wilde sort'. It was to be many decades before there was any reconciliation of the two 'sides'. Perhaps at the height of his popularity, Wilde actually felt he could effect a change in people's attitudes and he certainly did influence many, but often they were also homosexuals and he was, in a sense, preaching to an already converted audience. George Ives (1867–1950), a passionate campaigner against injustice faced by homosexuals, was absolutely bowled over and enthralled by Wilde when he met him, and Wilde in turn appreciated Ives's good looks, and they both had a desire to champion the idea of male beauty in the classical Greek sense. Ives had founded a secret homosexual society called The Order of Charonea, named after an ancient battle in which several hundred men had fought as one, bound together by ideas of friendship and love for each other. The idea of the nobility of men loving men no doubt created a common bond between Ives and Edward Carpenter too, as they were friends and met more than once.

One last effect of the Wilde trials should be mentioned. The trials would almost certainly have consolidated in the minds of many men – and some women – the nature of their unnamed and unspoken feelings for the same sex. Here was a man of art, money and status eloquently expressing feelings that they had too, and for many it must have been a 'road to

Damascus' moment. It may well even have led to some people finding the courage to seek out others like themselves, for companionship and affection. One must not make Oscar Wilde into any kind of martyr – he surely would have preferred to have been acquitted and gone back to his old life without hindrance, and in any case, unlike Radclyffe Hall some decades later, he did not intentionally enter the court rooms to stand as a leader of a cause, only to protect himself; as Wilde's biographer, Richard Ellman, wrote, at that time, society's 'Countenancing illegality did not amount to sanctioning it' and Wilde made the fatal mistake of thinking that he was so well liked that he was above the law. However, in bringing to public attention the complexities of opinion about same-sex love, Oscar Wilde's sacrifice was worth it if only because it brought some others to self-acceptance and knowledge; it was also a timely warning of the power of the law and that homosexual men needed to be very circumspect to stay the right side of that law. Further restrictions came into force in 1898 when 'cruising' public places such as the streets, parks, or public urinals, was criminalised as the offence of 'importuning' through the Vagrancy Act and the Criminal Law Amendment Bill. Importuning is to offer someone your services as a prostitute and should be seen as a different activity to what was later known as 'cottaging' when homosexual men met, often anonymously, at such places in order to have casual sex – although the law did not always see the nuances in their differences.

CHAPTER THREE

The Twentieth Century to 1957: The End of an Era

As Queen Victoria's long reign drew to a close, society's views on same-sex relationships were starting to shift. The growth of a campaign for women's rights including the vote, better-educated women – and prospects in the professions that were slowly opening up to them – enabled single women to earn better wages and to live independently in their own homes. However, these developments were beginning to make the male-dominated establishment uneasy. Women worked, or volunteered, in so many areas of life – from teaching to medicine, toiling on behalf of charities and poor-relief bodies, in their own businesses, and of course in the industrialised factory system. In 1901, 429,000 women were classified by the census return as in professional occupations, a four-fold increase over the latter half of the nineteenth century. Slowly, the idea of women having an intense same-sex friendship – whether the women were married or not – became a dubious thing, not something that kept them quiet and safe at home, and economic independence was seen by some as partly to blame for these unsavoury relationships.

The campaign that highlighted many of these trends was the movement demanding women's suffrage. In 1897 Millicent Fawcett had established the National Union of Women's Suffrage Societies and this was followed in 1905 by the Women's Social and Political Union (founded by Emmeline Pankhurst). Many women joined the cause, from all walks of life and levels of income. The fact that a high proportion of the women who joined these campaigns were unmarried and often forged close friendships with each other as they worked or even lodged together, has led to speculation among some historians that many were actively lesbian and may even have joined the campaigns in order to find same-sex relationships and that there is plenty of evidence, in diaries and other writings, that the women slept together on a regular basis. There are two issues to be addressed here. Firstly, it is more likely that single women would have had the time, money, and energy, to join a political campaign, while their married 'sisters' were more than likely hampered by children, domestic duties and a lack of funds. Being single does not necessarily imply homosexuality. Secondly, one has to bear in mind that in the late nineteenth century, it was extremely common to have to share a bed, either when visiting another house, or in one's own home due to domestic 'overpopulation'. Both genders and all age groups – and most social classes – had to do so at some point in their lives, and in some families and households, it was a nightly occurrence. Women such as Emily Wilding Davison (1872–1913), the militant campaigner who famously stepped in front of the king's horse at the Epsom Derby and sustained fatal injuries, and her inner circle of female friends, such as Mary Leigh, also a militant feminist campaigner, are obvious subjects for such a debate, but as historian Liz Stanley states, 'reading and interpreting the nature of this closeness is difficult indeed', and therefore one should not judge one way or the other beyond saying that they had a strong emotional bond, but that this was perhaps a part of their close political alliance too – comradely as much as romantic. Davison knew of Walt Whitman's poetry and owned a copy of his work; possibly love between 'comrades' would have been an acceptable way for her to show her feelings for other women. This is an extremely difficult theory to prove and is a good example of how two opposing sides can view relationships between women in a completely different way. Thus the fact that suffragettes sometimes shared a bed may or may not be significant. Ethel Smythe, composer of the suffrage anthem, had numerous affairs with women in her lifetime. However, to label all suffragettes as lesbian is a ridiculous as saying that all sailors are homosexual; some were, and some were not; some loved other women as comrades, but it went no further. One must, at all times in the history of sexuality, acknowledge a spectrum of feelings and actions.

One couple who certainly do seem to have been partners in every sense of the word are Edith (Edy) Craig (1869–1947) and Christabel Marshall (also known as Chris or Christopher St John, 1871–1960). Edy met Chris in 1899 when they were both working in theatre – Edy was the daughter of famous actress Ellen Terry. Despite a less than friendly first meeting, they were setting up home together within weeks and remained a devoted couple till Edy's death in 1947. As part of the women's suffrage movement, they kept an open house for women looking to hide from the police, or those needing a base to start again on release from prison.

The love affair between another campaigning couple, Eva Gore-Booth (1870–1926) and Esther Roper (1868–1938) was also to develop into a life-long partnership. At the time they met, Esther was established as the secretary of the North of England Society for Women's Suffrage, and was based in Manchester. Eva, who came from a wealthy Irish family, soon joined her love in the North of England and they committed to finding peaceful means of achieving the aims of the women's movement. They edited the *Women's Labour News* and went out of their way to encourage working-class women to join the suffrage movement, organising special campaigns for them and visiting them in their own homes; they can even be credited for encouraging Christabel Pankhurst to study law and join the women's suffrage movement, although their friendship with her was tarnished by their opposing views on the use of force – Eva and Esther wanted campaigns run by peaceful means only. By the time of the outbreak of war, Eva's health was delicate, but Esther was devotedly by her side until Eva died in 1926; Esther lived quietly as a 'widow' until her own death in 1938.

It was easier for women to set up home together if they had the financial means, as there were no laws restricting a lesbian relationship, and neighbours were just as likely to see them as companions for each other as a partnership in any other way. One positive that may have come out of the suffrage movement, and other women's campaigning groups, was that those of its organisers who were in same-sex relationships set an example to other women, showing that it was indeed possible to be yourself, love who you wished, and still live a successful and happy life. Some of these women will have been alienated from family, and others not, but at least they did not live with the fear of arrest as their homosexual 'brothers' did.

The 1901 census brought the continuing worry of public exposure and would have made men – and some women – living in the same household resort yet again to the usual evasions: describing their co-habiting lovers as boarders or lodgers, even as a relative or servant. To feel compelled to demean the most significant relationship in one's life by hiding it away so that the enumerator (often a local minister, teacher, or even police sergeant) would not have their attention drawn to anything 'untoward', must have been demoralising to say the least.

In 1905, psychoanalyst Sigmund Freud published *Three Essays on the Theory of Sexuality,* and it was his work – sometimes misinterpreted –

which took precedence as the medicalisation of homosexuality grew. He stated that homosexuals came about as a result of a combination of nature and nurture, and that had they developed 'normally', these men and women would have moved beyond the feelings they had for their own gender and matured into having a 'normal' sexuality. Why did this happen to some people and not others? Freud was unsure, but one of his theories – that of a combination of overbearing mother and weak father – was to influence generations of therapists, often to the great cost of their 'patients'. Today, Freud is often seen as the gremlin who led to the destructive treatment or 'cure' of many homosexuals, but at the time he was expounding his theories, he was never vitriolic about his subjects and in fact was more accepting than some, stating that homosexuals could *not* be cured, but what his disciples did with his ideas was more dangerous than he could have foreseen.

The legacy of Oscar Wilde lived on, either as a dire warning to homosexual men not to get caught, or as a shining example of all that was aesthetic and pure in same-sex attraction, and men continued to emulate him if they could. One such was Ronald Firbank (1886–1926), the writer, who was self consciously aesthetic, immaculately groomed in his loosely tailored suits, and never seen out without cane, bowler hat and gloves, not so unusual in those days, but add to this his face powder, lavish use of jewellery such as rings, a painfully thin physique and a rather flippant manner, and it was clear that here was no ordinary man. This was an image that Ronald created whilst a student at Cambridge, and it is reflected in his light-hearted stories. Even in the gaiety of the Edwardian era, men like Firbank would have stood out as different, whilst many working-class homosexuals, both male and female, would have gone out of their way to be discreet about their romances. However, everyone was to receive a sobering shock when the war started.

The First World War, 1914–1918

In 1914, a now iconic poster was produced that was to make its central figure even more famous than he already was. Lord Kitchener (1850–1916) is shown central to the poster, wearing a field marshall's cap and pointing directly at the viewer. The caption reads: 'BRITONS (Lord Kitchener) wants YOU … Join your country's army! God Save the King.' The central figure was by then a revered soldier who had made his name in the campaign to relieve Khartoum in the 1880s. As war began in 1914, Kitchener was appointed non-political secretary for war, and this, along with his popularity as a soldier, made him the ideal recruiting 'poster boy'. What the public cannot have known, however, was that Kitchener shared his home with his great love, Captain Oswald Fitzgerald, and had done for some ten years. This, no doubt, would have continued had they not both been tragically killed in the same naval disaster in 1916; the last sighting of them was of them talking together on the deck of their ship, which had been struck by a mine. Kitchener's body was never recovered.

Had Kitchener lived, perhaps his relationship with his partner would have been somehow leaked to the public, or at least whispered about in army circles, but dying so early in the war rendered him a hero and an iconic figure, his personal life remaining hidden from the grieving public at the time.

As they were illegal in civilian life, it almost goes without saying that homosexual acts were as frowned upon in the armed forces as in civil society. During the war, twenty-two officers and 270 enlisted men were court martialled for homosexual acts during the war. The Manual of Military Law contains the following passage in its chapter 'Acts of Indecency':

> It is a misdemeanour punishable with two years' imprisonment for any male person, either in public or in private, to commit or be a party to the commission of any act of gross indecency with another male person, or to attempt to procure the commission by any male person of any such act; and it is also a misdemean-our to do any grossly indecent act in a public place in the presence of more persons than one, or to publicly expose the person, or exhibit any disgusting object.

The punishment for sodomy was a minimum sentence of ten years and a maximum sentence of life. An officer found guilty of either crime would be discharged from the army without being sentenced; enlisted men did not receive such a reprieve.

The First World War is often seen as a time of liberation for women in Britain. Many kinds of employment were opened to them, including the armed services. After the war, some changes for women were sustained and others created. By 1928 the vote was made universal for all women over the age of 21. Women had better access to employment in the professions, the civil service, and to higher education. Clothing styles, more than likely influenced by the omnipresent military uniforms of the war, became more practical, tailored, and androgynous. Women had the opportunity to work in roles that had been almost completely closed to them before, such as the Ambulance division organised by Toupie Lowther (part of the First Aid Nursing Yeomanry), as bus conductresses (as they would have been known then), in the police, and in industries that desperately needed to replace the men they had lost from the shop floor. By 1918, 40,000 women were in the Women's Army Auxiliary Corps (WAAC), and in the same year the Women's Royal Air Force was founded. Others joined the newly established Women's Royal Naval Service, and undoubtedly there were women who were able to form discreet romantic attachments in these all female environments. One woman who was able to use the liberating effects of both access to the professions and the First World War to her advantage, was Lilian Barker (1874–1955; later Dame Lilian Barker). Born into the large family of a London tobacconist, she started her teaching career as a pupil teacher at her old school before attending teacher-training college in Chelsea. Later on she had to interrupt her teaching career to look after her invalid mother, but that was to prove a turning point rather than a setback – it was whilst she worked as a Sunday school teacher at this time that she met fellow teacher Florence Francis. Lilian and Florence were to be together till Lilian died in 1955. In 1914, after her mother died, 40-year-old Lilian moved in with Florence and her family – the first time she and the love of her life had lived under the same roof. Lilian began contributing to the war effort, teaching semaphore, signalling and cookery to women; she then went on to set up the cookery section of the Women's Legion. In 1916, she was appointed Superintendent of the Woolwich Arsenal, and it was she who had to effect the transition of the workforce to a female orientated one. By 1917, she was proud to announce that she had increased the female workforce to 30,000 from less than 100. Lilian also worked hard to provide money by fundraising for day nurseries and convalescent homes for the women workers, despite the fact that she regrettably could not do anything to improve their wages or working conditions. Such was the importance of her work that she was awarded the CBE. Lilian's career continued to flourish after the war, with Florence acting as home maker and driver for her partner, a long standing love that to the people Lilian helped, was immaterial, such was the support she gave to so many. The opportunities women like Lilian Barker offered to other women may well have compensated those who found that their same-sex feelings were increasingly being seen as a problem that needed addressing.

For men in the First World War, in the stinking trenches, underfed, lousy, and largely in poor condition before they ever got to the front, there was a pressing need for camaraderie and mutual support which undoubtedly resulted in a strong, even passionate friendships between men who were, in fact, only sexually attracted to women. One unlikely friendship resulted from the incapacity of soldier Fred Phillips who served in the Lancashire Fusiliers as a 'Bantam'. Standing 5ft tall in his socks, he was too short to serve in regular battalions and so joined one of the battalions especially created for smaller men who wanted to serve. He was gassed in the trenches in an enemy attack, and had severely congested lungs as a result but was still serving on the front lines till the end of the war. However, disabled by his poor breathing, he could not run away from danger like other men. His closest friend was another soldier who, at over 6ft tall, towered over his comrade. This unlikely pair became inseparable; the taller of the two even put his pal over his shoulder and carried him to safety when they were under fire, without doubt saving his life. Fred, who had done a few turns on the musical hall stages back in Blighty, buoyed his friend up with his irrepressible humour and his cheeky impersonations of officers (which lost him his corporal's stripe when an officer walked in on the show!), and together they struggled on to get through the war.

Fred never recovered from the damage to his lungs. Although he stuck it out to the bitter end of the war, and despite respite care at a convalescent home in North Wales, he was never able to hold down permanent work. He married and had three children, and his pal married too, but they never forgot each other and always kept in touch. When Fred died in 1940 of emphysema caused by the wartime mustard gas attack, his lanky friend attended the funeral, and cried like a baby at the loss of his beloved comrade. Fred's children, only school age at the time, never forgot the distress of this man who loved their father so much.

On a spectrum of same-sex bonds, where would this friendship lie? Born out of adversity, essential no doubt to their survival of that brutal conflict, this connection between the two men lasted until one died, and the survivor was devastated. There was no sexual element to their friendship, and more than likely one could not claim a romantic one either. Yet this close bond between two men in extreme circumstances can only be seen as a same-sex relationship, because clearly it is – today, it might be affectionately known as a 'bromance'. Looked at this way, the lines between platonic and romantic, deep friendships based on a mutual love, support, and need start to blur. They are different, and yet in many ways, the same. What is curious is that the commanders of the armed forces understood the need for such close bonds between comrades, and if they did not encourage it, would certainly not have looked askance upon them. Platonic love, affection and loyalty between soldiers was acceptable, but anything beyond that was a threat to discipline and downright treasonable.

As well as these close relationships forged by war, we have clear evidence of homosexual men and women finding relationships whilst serving their country. Siegfried Sassoon (1886–1967) and Wilfred Owen (1893–1918), both war poets of the finest calibre, were homosexual. Sassoon had a fine war record of great bravery and was awarded the Military Cross, but in 1916, partly because of the devastating death of his friend David Thomas, his stance changed and he began to oppose the war. Sassoon was one diarist who made reference to the sexual activity of other men on the front line, and expressed his attraction to soldiers he came across by chance – he was particularly taken with David Thomas and a teenage lad named Gibson, both of whom died in action. David Thomas is commemorated in various of Sassoon's poems such as *A Letter Home*:

> .... I've seen
> Soldier David dressed in green,
> Standing in a wood that swings
> To the madrigal he sings.
> He's come back, all mirth and glory,
> Like the prince in fairy story.

Towards the end of the war, in 1918, Member of Parliament Noel Pemberton Billing made the bizarre claim that German spies had compiled a list of 47,000 prominent English men and women who were engaging in homosexual activity and could be blackmailed by the Germans into helping the German war effort, the idea being that 'pillow talk' would cause a threat to the British war effort. He was to find himself the subject of a libel prosecution made by actress Maud Allen, whom he accused of being one of this dangerous crowd of sexual inverts. During the trial, which comes across in retrospect as a rather ridiculous and rowdy spectacle, poor Oscar Wilde was attacked yet again simply because it was his play that Maud Allen had been performing in. Both the judge and Lord Alfred Douglas, Wilde's former lover, denounced Wilde – now dead for the best part of nineteen years – as a filthy and perverting influence. Even after death, Wilde was seen as the enemy of respectability.

Also in 1918, the publisher of the book *Despised and Rejected* by A. T. Fitzroy found themselves in court, accused of making statements in the book (as publishers they took the responsibility) likely to prejudice the recruiting, training and discipline of persons in the armed forces – a contravention of the Defence of the Realm Act of 1914. Published in May of that year whilst the war was on-going, the book is of interest to historians of homosexuality as it deals almost equally with two groups who were on the fringes of society at the time – conscientious objectors, and homosexuals. In fact, the main male character, Dennis Blackwood, is both homosexual and a conscientious objector, and the lead female character is a young woman – Antoinette – who is lesbian but struggling to come to terms with her sexuality too. The two characters and their like-minded friends frequent Miss Mowbray's tea shop in London, known as a haunt of their 'kind', and it is partly through this viewpoint that we see the struggles, both personal and political, of the characters. The homosexual characters feel guilt and shame for being who they are, but at the same time the novel is used to point out to the reader that same-sex love is completely natural and normal to those who feel it. Dennis's lover tells him: 'For people made as we it's natural and beautiful to love as we love, and it's perversion in the true sense to try and force ourselves to love differently.' It is a touching and at times gruelling read, but empathy for the characters was in short supply in the media. James Douglas, who ten years later was to lead the vicious attack on the lesbian novel *The Well of Loneliness*, led the calls for Fitzroy's book to be withdrawn. The publisher, C. W. Daniel, was prosecuted and fined, and later published a condemnation of the novel: 'I would rather that any book were burnt than that I should be party to lending support to depravity of either the homo-sexual or the contra-sexual types' – he also claimed that the author had misled him into believing that the key same-sex relationship in the book was no more offensive than that of David and Jonathan, and that he only realised what it was all about when it was pointed out to him by others! As with *The Well of Loneliness,* it is likely that very few people would have read or been influenced by the book had others not made such a fuss about it (it only had a print run of just over 1,000 copies), but the related court case brought it to the attention of a much wider audience. Anyone reading the high-handed condemnations of the two themes, who also empathised with pacifism or were homosexual, would have thought twice about broadcasting their feelings to anyone else, especially as it came at a time when patriotism and conventionality were seen very much as the order of the day. It should be said as well that not all reviews of the book were entirely condemnatory – the *Times Literary Supplement* (TLS) of 22 May 1918 commented in its review:

> *The author's sympathy is plainly with the pacifists; and her plea for a more tolerant recognition of the fact that some people are, not of choice but by nature, abnormal in their affections is open and bold enough to rob the book of unpleasant suggestion. As a frank and sympathetic study of certain types of mind and character, it is of interest; but it is not to be recommended for general reading.*

This is a curious comment to make, suggesting that the author had a right to her empathy for the 'types' of people in the book and that she had done her job sensitively and well, but at the same time stating that perhaps the general public should be shielded from its influence.

The Post-War Conservative Backlash

It is possible that the harsh words about homosexuals towards the end of the war were a reaction to the liberating atmosphere that many people of all sexualities enjoyed at that time. Taken out of their home environment, the war had the same effect on the lives of some as waged labour and freedom to travel and live independently had had on others in the previous century. Another pleasing outcome of the war and the campaign for women's suffrage was that some women over the age of thirty were awarded the vote in 1919, a move designed to placate the women's movement and reward women for their contribution to the war effort. Naturally, not everyone approved of women being given the opportunity to express a political opinion via the ballot box and many thought they should return to their homes and children and carry on as before. Certain elements of the media and the establishment felt uneasy and threatened. This may be why there was an attempt in 1921 to make sexual relations between two women an offence under the 1885 Criminal Law Amendment Act, the act that tended to lump together restrictions on those seen as sexual deviants, and to protect the vulnerable from such people. The amendment was passed by 148 votes to 53 against in the House of Commons, but it was to fail in the House of Lords. It was first moved on 4 August by a Scottish Tory MP named Frederick McQuisten who, in his speech, lumped together drug addiction and neurological problems with lesbianism.

> *I know that to many Members of this House the mere idea of the suggestion of such a thing is entirely novel: they have never heard of it. But those who have had to engage either in medical or in legal practice know that every now and again one comes across these horrors* [lesbian relationships] ... *this horrid grossness of homosexual immorality should ... be grappled with .... it is only right that this House, which has the care of the law .... [should] do its best to stamp out an evil which is capable of sapping the highest and the best in civilisation.*

Another MP, Sir Ernest Wild, agreed, referring to a friend of his who was a nerve specialist: '... not a week passes that some unfortunate girl does not confess to him [the specialist] that she has been tampered with by a member of her own sex.'

Other MPs also contributed, making reference to debauchery, neurasthenia, vice, moral decline, and claiming that lesbianism was a cause of insanity, an undesirable obstacle to childbirth, and the result of abnormalities of the brain. A most peculiar form of opposition to the amendment came about when it was mooted that such a perversion should be kept quiet and not bandied about in acts of parliament – a former Director of Public Prosecutions warned: 'You are going to tell the whole world that there is such an offence, to bring it to the notice of women who have never even heard of it, never thought of it, never dreamed of it.' The Lord Chancellor concurred, adding his support by stating '... of every 1,000 women, 999 have never even heard a whisper of these practices.

CHAPTER THREE

Among all these ... the taint of this noxious and horrible suspicion is to be imparted.' This ridiculous reaction to the proposed amendment won the day thankfully, but is very telling in two areas: firstly, the implied weakness of mind and morals of all women, and the perceived predatory nature of lesbians. The idea that women were roaming the nation's newly built redbrick suburbs looking for other weak-willed women to violate is preposterous and the idea that their 'victims' had no strength of will to resist is just as bad. However, as sex reformer George Ives rightly pointed out, it was also the right decision because had women in homosexual relationships been criminalised alongside their male counterparts, they too would have possibly endured the misery and stress of blackmail, and at least women in same-sex relationships were spared that.

This view of the weak-willed housewife being preyed on by the predatory lesbian was widespread. Marie Stopes (1880–1958), who was a pioneer of family limitation, regarded lesbianism as a threat to the natural order of things – the heterosexual marriage. In her tract *Enduring Passions* (1923) she wrote:

> *Another practical solution which some deprived women find is in lesbian love with their own sex. The other, and quite correct name for what is euphemistically called lesbian love is homo-sexual vice. It is so much practised nowadays, particularly by the 'independent' type of woman, that I run the risk of being attacked if I call this thing by its correct name ... If a married women does this unnatural thing, she may find a growing disappointment in her husband and he may lose all natural power to play his proper part ... No woman who values the peace of her home and the love of her husband should yield to the wiles of the lesbian whatever the temptation to do so.*

There are a number of statements in this extract that are very telling. The first is the assumption that lesbians are predatory and will 'hunt down' and seduce – 'turn' – heterosexual women. This then leads, we are told, to the undermining of the marital relationship, emasculates the husband and could threaten a happy home. One or two responses to this are obvious. Firstly, society at the time assumed that all women were weak enough to be 'turned' lesbian and that their husbands would then be unable to satisfy them. Rather than being an attack on lesbianism, this sounds more like an advertisement for a same-sex seduction, not what the author intended at all! Secondly, there is a continuing emphasis on the idea that lesbianism is a perversion, something that Stopes was keen to convey because, as a eugenicist, she felt that homosexuality undermined marriage and hindered the development and creation of specially constructed families, which were robust in mind and body. There is also an oblique reference here to women who, after the tragic loss of men in the First World War, became part of a 'lost' generation of women of marriageable age who chose not to seek another partner once widowed, and led independent lives – sometimes sharing their home with another woman for economic and companionship reasons. Perhaps Stopes is assuming here that many of these women would end up indulging in 'homosexual vice' out of desperation and lack of a man to satisfy them, thus wasting their motherly instincts by lavishing them on a female instead of a child. Stopes was not the only person who may have viewed spinsters of childbearing age as suspect. Thanks to Freud's theory of arrested sexual development – that the pubescent crush with a member of the same sex was normal but something that most people grew out of, and homosexuals as congenitally abnormal people did not – many people pointed the finger of suspicion at single teachers and other female professionals at this time, and some researchers have seen this as nothing short of a campaign to undermine these intelligent, independent women. This is odd, as teaching was one of the professions seen in the Victorian era as acceptable for women to do because it employed their maternal instincts, so even if she was a spinster, a teacher was not 'wasting' her inborn gift for nurture. The nobility of motherhood and teaching – especially of younger children – was therefore entwined in some people's minds. Stopes could have backed up her claims with any number of works by 'experts'. A. C. Magian, a gynaecologist, wrote in his book *Sex Problems in Women* (1922) 'A confirmed tribadist is a most dangerous member of society ... usually a neurasthenic individual, irresponsible, hysterical and often mentally deranged' and goes on to describe lesbian relationships as 'violent attachments' which were deeply jealous to the point of violence. Many other publications condemned both female and male same-sex feelings to the same verbal destruction.

All this ruthlessly conventional thinking about family and sexuality is a far cry, however, from what Stopes was writing in her twenties whilst on an academic sabbatical in Tokyo. In February 1908, Stopes attended a ball

CHAPTER THREE

at the British Embassy, and was utterly captivated by the beautiful 'Mrs D', an American women whom Stopes thought was the most ravishing woman she had ever met. In her diary, after describing Mrs D's lovely ankles, white skin, gorgeous smile and gracious manner, she noted 'She is the only woman in Tokio [sic] who has bewitched me ...' and three days later she called on Mrs D by invitation:

> *I visited the charmer today, and stayed an unconscionably long time. No one has bewitched me in this way since my school days ... I had about half an hour of the Charmer to myself – her husband is the Naval Attache. She is simply alluring.*

Less than a week later, Stopes writes of taking tea with Mrs D: 'Why do I always fall in love with women?'

Bearing in mind that Stopes has mentioned schoolgirl 'crushes' it would not be surprising if any reader of this (which was published by Stopes in 1910 along with the rest of her journal from that time) saw it simply as a 'phase', a 'crush' or similar. Nevertheless, what she felt was a strong attraction to the other woman, and whether or not it was purely platonic or romantic is almost irrelevant, and clearly at the time she saw it as acceptable to publish these extracts as part of her record of her time in Tokyo. Perhaps the fact that she had these feelings outside the restrictive society of Britain made it seem less 'real' and more like a holiday romance.

However, in the 1930s the birth rate was falling whilst eugenicists like Stopes were keen to encourage not more, but 'better' families with fewer, carefully bred children of quality, and not only that, to have those families overseen and regulated by increasing state intervention. Spinsters may be teaching the next generation, but were not adding to it themselves, which was seen as another failure on their part, despite the fact that many local authorities insisted that teachers who married must resign, as their commitment was called into question. More criticism came from those who deplored the idea that women were teaching boys, which it was felt could undermine the masculinity of the next generation of men (a modernised repetition of the opinions expounded in the eighteenth century).

There is a big contradiction here. If these single teachers had had mainly male friends, then no doubt they would have been accused of being loose

93

women. If they had a circle of female friends, and worse still, shared their home with a woman for whatever reason, then they were perverts. Clearly the contempt for single women that had prevailed in Victorian times was alive and well decades later, and all this came against a background of greater media and public interest in 'inversion', wider freedoms for women in general, and even a change in the appearance of women, with more androgynous, practical, streamlined and tailored clothes. Teachers were being attacked with increasingly sexual references, and it was not uncommon for them to be referred to as 'man haters', and women who wished they had been born men, an accusation levelled at lesbians not only then, but in the present day too. It would certainly have been highly practical for a schoolteacher to wear the new streamlined clothes, but it came with a risk of facing accusations of 'mannishness'. What is worse is the idea that these embittered single women could also create a generation of similar young women moulded in their own likeness. Dr Williams, at an educational conference in 1935, was reported as saying that teachers of girls were 'embittered, sexless or homosexual hoydens who try to mould the girls into their own pattern' and furthermore these teachers were 'thin-lipped, flat chested, sadistic creatures.' The mannish title for some 1920s clothes was perhaps not without justification. At last, here genuinely were clothes that a female invert could wear that may better express her masculinity if she felt it, and thus give a signal to other women like herself that she was reaching out to make social or romantic contact. Author Radclyffe Hall, who was lesbian, had done her best as a young woman at the end of the Victorian era, toning down her clothes with their long skirts, hats and blouses to a puritanical tailored look with simple headwear and shirts and ties – not unknown on any woman who liked bicycling and tennis. However, by the time her lesbian novel *The Well of Loneliness* was published, she sported a short back and sides, men's shirts, and tailoring by men's tailors. This overtly male look was the sort emulated by many women who dared to try it in an effort – if not to build a lesbian community, to say 'I am here'. As Esther Newton puts it: 'Before they could find one another, they had to become visible, at least to each other.' Fashions were to become more flowing and feminine in the later 1930s, and as a result, those lesbians who retained a tailored, 'masculine' style of clothing stood out, and such outfits became more and more a way of presenting a masculine identity. At the end of the 1930s came another war, and a renewed opportunity to follow a trimmed-back

CHAPTER THREE

style again – and wear a uniform in many cases, and once again lesbians were more likely to 'blend in' rather than stand out.

Was the renewed pressure on women to be conventional a backlash against the advances made by the women's movement? By 1928, all women over the age of 21 had the right to vote. Many were in jobs that enabled independent living and more than that, were in professions that offered advancement and a real career. Thanks to the war, women had had the opportunity to see what it was like to work and have the camaraderie of the workplace; for many, the parental or marital home had been shown up for the lonely, suffocating places they could be. Perhaps accusing women of lesbianism was a convenient way to denigrate, humiliate and socially alienate any women who were beyond the control of their menfolk; and yet the attempt to make sexual acts between women an offence failed. There were plenty of other ways in society to keep women in their place without resorting to that, and the increasing growth of state interest in the family unit and the nation's children and their welfare, must have made single lesbians feel even more isolated, and determined to keep their private life exactly that, as private as possible. It is hardly surprising then that the publication of Radclyffe Hall's novel, *The Well of Loneliness*, was to cause such a sensation in 1928, bringing to public notice something that a male-dominated society had tried to keep covert. It was not the only novel that celebrated female independence and society at that time, but other novels did not receive the same condemnation. The 'Abbey' novels, aimed at young women – perhaps what we would in the twenty-first century refer to as 'Young Adult' novels – were a series of thirty-eight stories written by Elsie Jeanette Oxenham (1880–1960), beginning with *The Girls of the Hamlet Club* in 1914 and continuing right through to the 1950s. Various themes were included in the stories, but the author's intention was always to make better women out of her readers and any culturally aware novelist will adapt the themes in their books to reflect current opinions and matters of public interest. In 1928 Oxenham published *The Abbey Girls Win Through,* which includes a same-sex partnership between two women, Con and Norah. Con worked on the gloves counter in a large London store, and is described as the 'wife and home-maker', whilst 'Norah, the husband, planned little leisure trips and kept the accounts and took Con to the pictures.' Bearing in mind that this is very much a story for young girls, and in fact schoolgirls in gymslips are depicted on the dust wrapper of the first edition, this must be reflecting a domestic arrangement that a good proportion of the readership may have encountered in their neighbourhood. Whether for reasons of practicality, romance or anything else, female same-sex households were an accepted feature of the times, but when they were explicitly labelled as inverted or lesbian, then it suddenly became unacceptable and the women involved, persona non grata.

It is no surprise, bearing in mind the continued pressure on women at this time to be conventional, married and feminine, that some women still felt the need to cross dress in order to conceal their same-sex relationships – or to be able to support a 'wife' on a man's wage at a time when disparity in pay was so marked. In 1929, what looks like a classic 'female husband' news story was published in the *Daily Herald* of 10 May:

> *The discovery was made when a person, giving the name of William Sidney Holton, aged 42, timber carrier ... was admitted to Evesham Poor Law Infirmary, where she now lies dangerously ill ... it is stated that for four and a half years she has lived with another woman, and posed as this woman's husband. This statement is corroborated by the supposed wife, a single woman, aged 31, of Birmingham, who met Holton when 'he' was working at her brother's coal wharf in Birmingham. 'He' was then living with a woman.*

Holton's wife then went on to say that she never had any suspicions about her new lover who always seemed to be very strong and who 'smoked from two to three ounces of tobacco weekly in a clay pipe'; Holton eventually lived with the young woman as a couple and took on the woman's young child as her own. Some time afterwards, the 'wife' had another baby and on the birth certificate Holton is declared to be the father, an act that constituted an offence because it was a false declaration. When Holton's gender was revealed due to her illness, the wife was prosecuted for doing this and it was a rare occasion when Holton appeared at the trial in female attire, in fact it was thought it was the first time in twenty years.

Many of the women who were able to live openly as homosexual both during and after the war had independent means and an existing public profile – Radclyffe Hall, Toupie Lowther, Mary Allen and Lady Una Troubridge are only four examples. The vast majority of research so far has concentrated on these high profile women, almost as if by showing

CHAPTER THREE

they had such freedoms, then all female inverts did. Can a sexually and culturally liberated life have been possible for all female inverts, especially those without social and financial freedom? When *The Well of Loneliness* was published in 1928, the author, Radclyffe Hall, used her considerable wealth and social position to live her life as she chose and therefore had an advantage over poorer or disadvantaged women, many of whom had to marry for security and to conceal their sexuality. A well known (although not particularly popular) figure on the London social scene and in artistic lesbian circles in Paris – as author Diana Souhami puts it, Hall 'had an awesome sense of her own importance' – Hall was living with Lady Una Troubridge in what they both regarded as a marriage, and indeed she put great emphasis on her high-profile relationship as an example of how same-sex couples could be devoted exclusively to each other in the long term – in other words, her lesbian marriage should be regarded in that sense as being as valid as that between a man and a woman (very much along the lines of what Havelock Ellis saw as a 'normal' lesbian relationship) and an example to others of her kind who wanted to embark upon a long term relationship. By 1928, Hall's career was at its height. She was a popular novelist, with her most recent novel, *Adam's Breed*, published in 1926 to great acclaim and lively sales; for this novel she won the Prix Femina literary prize and also the James Tait Black prize. For some years Hall had been planning a book that would be a sympathetic portrayal of homosexuality, but she had been biding her time until her popularity was at its greatest so that the story would reach the largest and most receptive audience. This was not a book aimed only at other homosexuals – it was her avowed mission to educate the public, and it was a mission that she took very seriously indeed. The story – which Hall was at great pains to say was not autobiographical – follows the life of Stephen Gordon, a masculine lesbian whose persona owes much to the image of the masculine inverted female as first described by Kraft–Ebing and Havelock Ellis. Stephen's difficult yet privileged early life is followed by a series of doomed lesbian love affairs and then it is directly linked to the liberating influences of the First World War as she volunteers to drive ambulances for the war effort, wears a uniform, and meets her female lover, the gentle Mary, whilst doing this. Following the template of *The Unlit Lamp*, Stephen also needed to get away from home to live a fulfilled life and express herself fully through her sexuality – another reason why the book may have been seen as dangerous to women and to families; she

97

was also very masculine in her mannerisms, physical build and manner of dress (and there are similarities to the female husbands of old here). Hall was keen to represent her key characters as having been born with the potential for same-sex desires, something that could not be helped; essentially the book was a plea for acceptance for something that was innate and therefore to that individual, natural. It could be argued that even for its times, the novel was admirably restrained; the closest the narrative gets to anything remotely sexual were the famous phrases 'and that night, they were not divided'; and 'she kissed her full on the lips'.

The imagery of poisons that was prevalent in the beginnings of the Obscene Publications Act in 1857 returned with a vengeance to haunt Hall and her book. On Sunday 19 August 1928, just as Jonathan Cape published the novel, editor James Douglas (a veteran anti-book campaigner who had led the criticism of the novel *Despised and Rejected*) launched a vicious campaign against *The Well*, stating famously in his editorial entitled: 'A Book That Must be Suppressed':

> *I am well aware that sexual inversion and perversion are horrors which exist amongst us today ... I have seen the plague stalking shamelessly through great social assemblies, I have heard it whispered about by young men and women who do not and cannot grasp its unutterable putrefaction ... It is no use to say that the novel possesses "fine qualities", or that it's author is an "accomplished" artist. It is no defence to say that the author is sincere, or that she is frank, or that there is delicacy in her art ... It* [the novel] *is a deductive and insidious piece of special pleading designed to display perverted decadence as a martyrdom inflicted upon these outcasts by a cruel society ...*
>
> *I would rather give a healthy boy or a healthy girl a phial of prussic acid than this novel. Poison kills the body, but moral poison kills the soul. What, then, is to be done? The book must at once be withdrawn ...*
>
> *Fiction of this type is an injury to good literature ... Literature has not yet recovered from the harm done to it by the Oscar Wilde scandal.*

Here again one must reflect on the impact of the news story on its readership, whatever their sexuality. The idea of poison being more preferable than association with any literature which even mentioned same-sex attraction must have shocked and frightened many, and as the reading public is easily impressed by what the mass media says, the opinions of many must have been affected by this. Worse was to come. In an act that was to infuriate and dismay Hall, especially as sales of the book were rising, her publisher sent the book to the Home Secretary, Sir William Joynson-Hicks (a Christian fundamentalist), along with some reviews, and also invited its perusal by the Director of Public Prosecutions. The end result was a trial in which the Hicklin test was applied to see how offensive the book was; the book was duly banned and an appeal failed to overturn the decision. To compound the insult, the judge, Sir Charles Biron, conceded that the book was even more dangerous because it was well written, and the appeal judge, Sir Robert Wallace, denounced the novel as obscene, disgusting, dangerous and corrupting. The impact of the trial must have been a mixed blessing for other lesbians, pretty much all of whom were Hall's inferiors socially and financially; some must have been frightened by the publicity their sisterhood was receiving, and far from giving them confidence, it may well have made them even more covert in their expressions of their sexuality or prevented them from expressing it at all.

The irony of it is that Hall's previous novel, *The Unlit Lamp* (1924), which had a powerful female same-sex theme in it and also critiques the claustrophobic home life of many middle-class girls and women (and it even includes a rather dubious relationship between a key character and her mother), passed completely unnoticed, possibly because the two women who planned to move away and live together have something of a passionate friendship about them rather than an overtly sexual desire. It also has something of a feminist theme in the way the tentacles of home and family life clung on to girls and women, stifling their individuality and education – in fact the original title was *Octopus*. It is a better written book than *The Well of Loneliness*, but because the latter was the flagship of Hall's great crusade, it received all the attention. The women who had had undreamt of freedoms in the First World War may well be struggling to keep them as a stronger sense of 'normality' returned to the country. However, women who were living together purely because they had no husband or their man had died in the war – a convenient arrangement for economic purposes, independence and companionship – must have worried that people would look askance at them and see their friendship in a new light. Feminist commentators have a specific interpretation of these households and other all female groups. If one takes Adrienne Rich's theory of the 'lesbian continuum', any group or household of women living together could be seen as a lesbian arrangement in that it is all female, which broadens out the idea of lesbianism to include a huge range of situations. Indeed, any woman, married (to a man) or otherwise, can be seen as lesbian if she is involved in an emotional, sexual, or political commitment to other women. In fact, it could be said that if one takes a broad enough view, this community-based theory of sisterhood sees *all* women as lesbian. It is a very appealing and a liberating concept to have a definition for a group of women that encompasses affection, love, sisterhood and support. It also takes the word 'lesbian' out of a strictly sexual or romantic connotation and gives it many more dimensions. If two or women live together perfectly amicably, without any attraction towards each other beyond friendship and co-operation, and that is seen as a lesbian arrangement, all danger and condemnation is taken out of the word. However, this would have been no consolation to the women who felt uneasy in 1928 as the trial of *The Well* unfolded, and of course, after the court case, Hall could go back to her affluent life and loves and just carry on, even if her pride had been wounded.

The novel has been criticised by late twentieth century commentators for its reinforcement of a 'butch–femme' dynamic, that is, what looks like a role play of a heterosexual marriage with a 'wife' (the femme) and a 'husband' (the butch or more dominant masculine partner), which the radical feminist movement of the 1970s was to reject as being a reflection of patriarchal domination, and even at the time the novel was published it baffled many lesbians who could not recognise themselves in either of these roles. However, admirers of Hall flocked to see her at the courtroom during the trial, and pressed forward to greet her outside, kissing her hand and applauding her, all of which reinforced Hall's conviction that she had done the right thing in publishing the book. Hall also received hundreds of letters from lesbians thanking her for making them feel less alone, and less like an isolated and unique freak of nature. Although bitterly disappointed by the ban, she was aware that the book was still available covertly in Britain, thanks to the publisher Pegasus Press who printed it in Paris; it also remained openly on sale in the USA. In 1949,

CHAPTER THREE

Una Troubridge negotiated a reprint of all Hall's fiction via Falcon Press, decent quality volumes that are readily available to buy today, and this included *The Well of Loneliness*. No challenge was made to its inclusion and it is now widely available in a variety of formats, including for e-readers.

Despite the fact that *The Well of Loneliness* is virtually the only novel that Hall is remembered for today, she did write some other commendable works, including, of course, *The Unlit Lamp*, and the short story, *Miss Ogilvy Finds Herself*, which also address issues of sexuality and the difficulties of expressing it in Hall's lifetime.

The long-term impact of *The Well of Loneliness* should not be underestimated. It may not have been the best piece of fiction Hall ever produced, and there were plenty of other novels with lesbian themes on the market at the same time which escaped the condemnation *The Well* faced, but then Hall had deliberately challenged the establishment with her book and was an out and proud masculine lesbian who, in many ways defied convention in her own lifestyle. Plenty of copies of the book circulated in Britain, and even in the 1950s, women found it of great comfort to know through reading the book that they were in fact part of a group in society who felt just like they did. Hall's descriptions of a homosexual community of sorts, with its own social venues (even if in the story they are in Paris), the image of Stephen and Mary living in domestic harmony, and the very thought that 'out there' are people just like you that you could reach out to, was a revelation to many women and probably some men too. As flawed as the book is, it brought the incalculable gift of hope.

Some historians of female homosexuality cite the above factors as being positive steps towards if not the emancipation of female inverts, then their realisation that they had an identity, and one which they could seek to recognise in other women in order to make social and support contacts or even networks. Judith Halberstam has cautiously pointed out common ground between nineteenth century tribades and female husbands, the inter-war female invert, and later representations of the post Second World War 'butch' lesbians, almost suggesting a positive continuum of the development of lesbian identity. It would not have felt like that if one was a single woman living through the difficult inter-war years, but it is a pleasing theory nonetheless which suggests some long-term improvement for female homosexuals.

Popular Culture

The majority of people who watched the plays, musicals and movies of the inter-war period were completely unaware that many of their favourite songs or scenes were created by homosexual men and some women. Noel Coward (1899–1973) was one of the best known and most popular theatre figures in Britain. His wit, suave appearance characterised by silver cigarette holders and immaculate evening wear, and his seemingly upper class, clipped way of speaking (which was actually developed in an effort to communicate with his deaf mother!) became his trademarks, but he was never open with the public about his sexuality, which would have been the death of his career at the time. He did enjoy playing with his audiences, however, and in his song 'Green Carnation' made fun of the young male followers of Oscar Wilde who wore a green carnation like him and were equally 'aesthetic' in their manners and preferences. Cardiff born Ivor Novello (David Ivor Davies, 1893–1951) was also hugely popular, with his musicals *Glamorous Night* and *Dancing Years* delighting packed theatres, yet even in his 1951 biography by W. Macqueen-Pope, *Ivor: the story of an achievement,* there is little to indicate his private life. How would those who disapproved of same-sex love have felt, to know that one of their favourite songwriters, who had penned the wildly successful song of the First World War, *Keep the Home Fires Burning,* was in fact homosexual? Two years after writing this song, Ivor met his long-term companion, actor Bobby Andrews, and they remained together for thirty-five years and even both performed in some of Ivor's musicals. Not all celebrities coped well, either with their sexuality or with having to conceal it – British actor Charles Laughton (1899–1962) struggled to come to terms with his feelings, which he revealed to his wife, actress Elsa Lanchester, in 1930 when they had been married a year. His homosexuality was widely known amongst his fellow actors and of no consequence to them, but he was tormented by it, and one wonders if life would have been easier for him if the law had been different and openness was acceptable.

Equally, the literary reading public who enthused over the works of Virginia Woolf (1882–1941) and the other members of the renowned Bloomsbury Set had no idea that these authors and artists were leading highly unconventional private lives, and that included homosexual relationships. In December 1922, Virginia Woolf met Vita Sackville-West (1892–1962) and had an affair with her; she was enamoured enough to write *Orlando*, a fantastical tale of time travel and gender swapping published in 1928 (the same year as *The Well of Loneliness,* but perhaps because it was regarded as 'literary' and not 'popular' fiction it was more favourably received) and based on the persona of her lover. In a letter to Vita as she started work on the story, Virginia wrote '… suppose Orlando turns out to be Vita; and it's all about you and the lusts of your flesh and the lure of your mind … shall you mind?' – a phrase Vita was to cautiously omit from a radio broadcast in which she read out the letter, many years later, to maintain the privacy of their love for each other and the real reason for the writing of the book. Only those who knew the two women would have guessed that it had been inspired by their largely romantic love affair and was really an adoring portrait of Vita. The writer E. M. Forster, who was a close friend of Woolf's, would not allow his same-sex themed novel *Maurice* to be published in his lifetime, and as a result his writing career flourished and he was a popular literary figure. The public would have been horrified to find out that he did have affairs with other men; for example the policeman Bob Buckingham, whom he met at a friend's house, provided Forster with a romance which may have been physical, but was also a close friendship that survived Bob's marriage and lasted till Forster's death (he actually passed away in the Buckingham household). Vita Sackville-West had already caused scandal by eloping several times with her childhood love, Violet Trefusis, starting in 1918. They frequently went to France where they would promenade the Parisian boulevards with Vita dressed as a male, and playing the chivalrous beau to the hilt, to Violet's more feminine persona. Eventually their distraught husbands both travelled to beseech them to end the affair for the sake of the marriages and family honour. Vita's husband was fellow invert Harold Nicholson, and they had an open relationship as he too had same-sex affairs, but the violence of Vita's feelings for Violet threatened this amicable marital arrangement. Whilst they were lovers, the two young women kept up a flow of passionate letters to each other of which sadly only Violet's to Vita survive; Violet was not able to keep Vita's letters as her jealous husband demanded that she destroy them. Here is an example of a letter written by Violet to Vita, on 3 March 1920:

I want you so, Mitya [Violet's pet name for Vita]. *I lie awake for hours at night, longing for you hungrily, hopelessly … if you ceased to care for me, I should cease to live … Never say I don't love you, if I have to travel across Europe sitting bolt upright, to England which I detest, braving the fury of my mother, merely to catch a glimpse of you! Je t'adore ...*

And later on 11 May 1920:

... I have been ardently wishing we were ten years older; then people wouldn't care what we did or where we went – or even twenty years older. I don't care how old I am provided I may be with you ... Ever since I was a child I have loved you. Lesser loves have greater rewards – You don't know what you have been – what you are to me: just the force of life, just the raison d'etre ... Somewhere, tucked away in the recesses of your nature, there is something which understands – something which responds to my touch like a harp string – something alien, and wild, and uncouth – something savage and untender, something fiercely willing, and fiercely hostile to the rest of you.

After Vita's death in 1962, her son found a manuscript written in a notebook describing the passionate affair with Violet, and ten years later it was published. This, in many ways, makes up for the loss of Vita's letters – we read that Vita, in her words, looked like a 'rather untidy young man ... in Paris I practically lived that role. Violet used to call me Julian.' She wrote that in September of 1920 '... the whole of that Summer she was mine – a mad and irresponsible Summer of moon light nights, and infinite escapades, and passionate letters, and music, and poetry ... things weren't tragic, they were rapturous and new, and one side of my life was opened to me ...'

Very few affairs can continue at that level of intensity and the two women eventually went their separate ways. Violet became a feted literary hostess and writer residing in Paris, and Vita turned to family life in the form of her two sons and her husband, and also built a career as a poet and novelist. They stayed in regular contact and Violet would stay at Vita's home, Sissinghurst; one of her sons recalled how charismatic and intriguing Violet was, and how she used to study the two boys as if they were some kind of strange curiosity. The close bond between the women remained, albeit in a different form, although at times it seemed that those passionate feelings were still there, simmering, and simply awaiting an opportunity to overflow again. After one of Violet's visits to Sissinghurst in the early 1940s, Vita wrote to her: 'I don't want to fall in love with you all over again … my quiet life is dear to me … But if you really want me, I will come to you always, anywhere'.

By the 1950s things had settled down into a deep attachment. Vita now wrote to Violet: 'The time when we were in love has gone by, leaving us with this queer deep love … There is a very queer thing between you and me, Lushka [her pet name for Violet]. There always was.' Vita died in 1962, Violet in 1972, and it was not until after they had both gone that their passionate words came into the public domain. Violet and Vita were privileged and accomplished, but their passion could have been replicated across the social strata – why should not two women who worked in a shop or a factory feel as they did, want to escape together and risk all for a chance to be as one? Poor and working-class women may not have written down their feelings for each other, but the feelings would have been there nonetheless.

T. E. Lawrence published an abridged subscriber's edition of his book *The Seven Pillars of Wisdom* in 1926; it is dedicated to 'S.A.' who is now widely thought to be Salim Achmed, a young man whom Lawrence was very close to but who died aged 19 in 1919. In 1936, poet W. H. Auden wrote the famous poems to accompany the popular *Night Train* films made to show the work of the Post Office, which quickly became iconic pieces of documentary film making and made Auden a household name; Auden was at the time in a long-term relationship with New Yorker Chester Kallman, a partnership that was to last until Auden's death in 1973. It is highly unlikely that many of the cinema-going public knew anything of Auden's personal life.

The author Naomi 'Mickie' Jacob (1884–1964), a popular and financially successful writer in the 1920s and 1930s, was overtly masculine with her cropped hair, tailored suits and predilection for coarse 'tap room' jokes, but as she lived abroad for reasons of her health she was rarely seen on the London literary scene. She never watered down her appearance though, and any photograph of her in the English newspapers would have made her stand out as different. Somehow the reading public managed to ignore it however, presumably thinking it was all part of the eccentricity of the artiste, and because they enjoyed her books. It was always easier to plead aesthetic eccentricity and get away with looking 'queer', than for a working-class woman or man to do the same.

In the cinemas, audiences thrilled first to the silent movies and then to the 'talkies' after that. Did they ever guess that some of their favourite stars were in fact involved with lovers of the same gender? The list is long: silent stars Alla Nazimova, Josephine Hutchinson and Ramon Novarro, major stars such as Greta Garbo, and Marlene Dietrich played vamps, heroes and housewives, nearly always looked glamorous (whether in gowns or masculine tailoring), and in real life were often in marriages arranged by their film studio to keep any rumours at bay. Silent movie heart throb Rudolph Valentino was married off twice in what were known as 'lavender marriages' – that is, designed as a cover for homosexual artistes – to Jean Acker (1920) and Natacha Rambova (1923; a former lover of Alla Nazimova), who both had lesbian relationships, and although there were spiteful comments in the press about Valentino's effeminacy – in 1926 the *Chicago Tribune* lambasted Valentino as a 'painted pansy' – his fans more than likely chose to think otherwise, and after his untimely death in the same year, more than 100,000 grief-stricken women crowded his funeral and there were equal levels of dismay in Britain. It was more than an actor's career was worth to reveal their true feelings, because it could mean the end of that career.

If these public figures were not able to show their true feelings for each other, express their feelings for partners and close friends honestly and openly, and did not want to be a model of behaviour for anyone else like them for fear of public humiliation and loss of income, then there were no role models for homosexuals within public life to look up to. Why did these influential people not stand up as Radclyffe Hall did, and speak for their own same-sex 'family'? Some would certainly have feared the loss of income and prestige; others would have wished to protect their partners from scrutiny, and of course the men had to fear the wrath of the law. Their creative output was sometimes cautious, almost like a form of self-censorship, not just of their art but of their own sexuality. The best they could do was to scatter some 'in' jokes throughout their work for like-minded people to pick up on. There were songs like *Green Carnation* to enjoy, but many will have avoided any comment about it to friends and family. Just like their media idols, they feared exposure and condemnation, but that meant a big secret was lying heavy in their hearts, eating away at them. It is hard to live as someone you are not, and late twentieth century studies have shown unequivocally that there are huge psychological and physical benefits to 'coming out' as homosexual, benefits that were denied to all but a minority earlier in the century.

CHAPTER THREE

The Beginnings of a Homosexual Social Network

If this claustrophobic life was the norm, how did ordinary homosexual men and women in the 1920s and 1930s meet other people like themselves, and find lovers or even life partners? It was extremely difficult unless you lived in an urban area, specifically a city such as London, to find any networks at all. In London, however, a homosexual sub-culture – hardly a community, but definitely a network – continued to grow slowly but surely. The Trocadero and the Cavour Bar in Leicester Square, the Golden Lion in Soho, and the Running Horse in Mayfair (mixed men and women) were known 'friendly' social haunts. Certain areas were known to be useful for meeting up, and certain signals such as wearing a particular colour (such as mauve or purple) or a certain type of shoe (suede) or garment (camel hair coats, or a particular colour of shirt), and ways of addressing another person were a form of 'code'. Jewellery could be significant, such as a ring worn on the little finger of the left hand of a lesbian. Thus, like a rainbow coloured wristband today, these signals were a safe way of identifying a friendly associate or potential partner. Those who were more daring would pass as the other gender – so a woman might wear male tailoring and have her hair in a severe crop – and men may wear cosmetics and feminine accessories, as did the flamboyant Quentin Crisp. Assignations could happen at certain public toilets or other venues such as public houses, and male prostitutes could be found in the West End and a number of shopping thoroughfares. Naturally, people in the provinces had desires and feelings too. Simon, a gentleman who grew up in the Midlands in the inter-war years, described how he would 'meet' other men for the first time:

> *You would just be walking along and then a chap who looked nice would go past, and I would think "Ooh I like the look of him," and you would catch his eye and give him a 'look', and if he did the same back, you might turn round and follow him and have a chat, and take it from there. It was all you could do really, and you had to be careful!*

Simon was married; he revealed his homosexuality to his wife and she stood by him throughout a marriage lasting several decades, never giving up his secret to the day she died. Simon's two children also never knew about their father's sexuality, although:

I think my nephew guessed, but he never said anything to my wife or kids. But he did keep his children away from me, my great nieces and nephews. That hurt my feelings, it was as if he was secretly saying that I would prey on them. That was so upsetting.

It is little wonder that men like Simon would be cautious in finding partners. Between 1918 and 1939, there were about 700 arrests per year in Britain for homosexual offences, with a noticeable rise from the early 1930s onwards (299 reported offences of indecency between men, 1935–39), and the danger of blackmail was everywhere there were homosexual men looking for affection or a casual liaison. In the late 1930s a blackmail gang consisting of one Harry Raymond and eleven other males – some known to the police as sodomites – was arrested for its activities, not just in London but as far afield as Cornwall and the Shetland Islands. The modus operandi was for a young man of their group – usually an older teenager – to approach an older man who looked to be of good social standing, and allow the man to enact a trivial sexual act with him in exchange for a small amount of money. This continued over a period of time and then another slightly older male contacted the victim, posing as a concerned older brother. He tells the victim that money is needed to get the little brother away from that sort of life and so the demands for cash began, anything from £50 to thousands of pounds being handed over. Harry Raymond (a former actor whose real name was Arthur Clive Gould) seems to have been the mastermind of this racket and he was eventually prosecuted at the Central Criminal Court and sent to prison.

Understandably, for many, private parties and 'clubs' were preferable to socialising or 'cruising' in public places. However, even at a private event one was not always safe. In 1933, police infiltrated a house party at which homosexual men and women were socialising, some of the men cross dressing, some guests dancing and generally enjoying the event. At least thirty people who had attended the party were charged with conspiracy to corrupt morals and keeping a disorderly house.

Some venues were a little less circumspect in hosting their diverse clientele. As early as 1912, Madame Strindberg's The Cave of the Golden Calf opened in Heddon Street, off Regent Street in London, and is now regarded as the first 'gay pub'. The Caravan Club in Endell Street in the centre of London prided itself on its bohemian customer base, which included lesbians, homosexuals (some of whom were apparently prostitutes), and people of colour. The club boldly promised 'all night gaiety' at the 'most unconventional spot in town', but such boldness came at a price – numerous prosecutions as a disorderly house through the 1930s and even into the first years of the Second World War. At one notorious trial in 1934, the packed courtroom heard that this venue allowed men to embrace in a romantic manner and to cross dress and behave in a female way, and that lewd behaviour was commonplace. There are shades of the masked ball in Hulme in 1880 in this venue – many of the defendants were young men and their occupations suggest a mixture of working class and professional – artist, window dresser, waiter, messenger, dancing partner, painter, school master, traveller, milliner, clerk, and salesman. The judge, Mr Henry Holman Gregory KC, denounced the place as 'A foul den of iniquity' and point-blank refused to allow one of the defendants to demonstrate the rumba in the courtroom! Other places also offered a relatively safe venue (until raided by the police) for these same minority groups – the Running Horse public house, and Billie's Club (in Denmark Street in Soho) also hosted a similar mix of people and were prosecuted in the same way. These venues demonstrate a necessity for certain minority groups to have a place to socialise in peace without being stared at, abused, or even attacked, and presumably the homosexual and racial minorities amicably shared their safe spaces on the basis of there being some safety in numbers. For those who wanted a more everyday meeting place, certain Lyon's tea houses were known as gathering points, and Quentin Crisp, the flamboyant homosexual whose life as a young queer man in London was famously dramatised in the 1970s, patronised the Chat Noir café in Old Compton Street with his homosexual friends.

There is one aspect of community cohesion that Simon certainly knew of, although whether he had the chance to use it in a provincial town is doubtful. That is Polari, the 'secret' language used by homosexuals in the twentieth century, which only started falling into disuse in the 1960s. Polari is a slang language, often changing and evolving, that was used by circus folk, sailors and others, long before it was adopted and became known as a 'gay' language. It gained its vocabulary from many sources, including Romani, Yiddish, London slang, and Italian, reversed words (riah for hair, for example) and it was a safe way to talk to another homosexual without 'outsiders' knowing what you were saying. Some words would be familiar, such as 'bevvy' for a drink, but others, such as 'Brenda' or 'friend of Brenda' were unique – that means the person is a police officer, someone definitely to be wary of if you were out and about with homosexual friends! Here is an example: 'Vada the bona ome with the blue ogles? He's on the national handbag!' This translates as 'See the nice looking man with the blue eyes? He's on the dole!' 'Bona ome' was also widely used as the Polari phrase for homosexual.

Polari was later popularised by comedian Kenneth Williams in the hit radio series *Round the Horne* (1965–1968), with his gloriously camp characters Julian and Sandy. They usually cropped up in a sketch when Kenneth Horne, their straight man in the programme, happened upon them in all innocence, and they invariably introduced themselves with 'Hello, I'm Julian and this is my friend Sandy!' Their repartee would follow, with very generous references to Polari along the way. Julian and Sandy seemed to drift from one enterprise to another, each week with a different business, such as Bona Pets. Outrageous double entendres would be put into the Polari-filled dialogue, often going unnoticed because nobody really knew what Julian and Sandy were talking about! On a more serious level, Polari had some very valuable uses. It gave homosexual men a common parlance, and one which gave them the privacy to speak about forbidden topics in public places because most people would not understand them; and if a homosexual man heard the slang being spoken, he would know perhaps that he was in a safe venue and could socialise with more ease than he would normally.

Despite these promising beginnings of a homosexual network of sorts, some aspects of communication continued to be woefully slow to develop. One magazine for women that grew out of the culture of the Suffrage movement with its higher proportion of feminist allies, was *Urania*. This curious journal, with a circulation of only a few hundred, championed a complete rethink of gender and sexuality boundaries, and like their Victorian foremothers, the editors saw a close, almost spiritual bond between women as the ideal relationship. Eva Gore-Booth was one activist who wrote for the journal and believed passionately in its campaign to throw off the shackles of gender roles. In this sense they rejected the, by then, largely accepted theory of inversion where a homosexual man had a woman's soul and vice versa. Although not overtly about lesbianism, it did cover many stories about cross-dressing

110

women, same-sex marriages and so on, and historian Alison Oram has suggested it was read mainly by women from the Suffrage movement itself. It lasted from 1916 to 1940 when it seems that its readership got so small – they were literally dying out and not being replaced by a younger readership, despite trying its best to recruit new readers in the 1920s – that it was no longer worthwhile, but even at its height it is unlikely to have reached any women outside those rather exclusive circles. For men, there was but one issue of *The Quorum: a magazine of friendship,* privately published in 1920. It offered poems and short stories about friendship between men, and was produced by the Order of Chaeronea, a secret homosexual society set up in the 1890s.

Also, during the inter-war years, there continued to be a link made between homosexuality and extreme left wing politics, or Communism. A group of communist sympathisers that comprised intellectuals such as W. H. Auden and Christopher Isherwood (both homosexual) became known as the 'homintern', a play on words as the shortened version of the movement Communist International was 'Comintern'.

From a psychiatric point of view, homosexuals continued to be classed as suffering from some form of illness or psychological 'deformity' and the 'mind doctors' were still working hard to make their reputations by finding a cause for it (because if there is a cause, there must be a cure). One very typical book of the inter-war years is *Strange Lust* by Dr Angelo Louis Marie Hesnard (1886–1969), published in 1933 in English translation; Hesnard is regarded as an important figure in French sexology studies and as such his pronouncements were taken very seriously. Hesnard lists a baffling array of possibilities as the causes of homosexuality:

- Infantile sexual dreams.
- Excessive self abuse, when conducted for its own sake and not for 'normal sexual satisfaction' may 'unquestionably' lead eventually to homosexual behaviour.
- General organic conditions created by the endocrine glands 'which undoubtedly exists as the basis of all definite homosexuality. We can find proof of this in the frequent physical resemblance, (and) in temperament, between the homosexual and his mother'.
- Ordinary organic causes such as hereditary syphilis toxic infection, or dreams in embryo or in childhood.

111

- Alcohol abuse in the adult 'renders a person salacious and more perverted in different ways, even where there is no recognisable disposition' (to homosexuality).
- Age: 'certain latent homosexuals or bisexuals only become homosexuals … at a late date, at a time when their sexual potency is weakest.'
- Psychopathic and mentally unbalanced patients demonstrate a 'curious alteration' from heterosexual to homosexual desires.
- Practice makes perfect! Anyone who practises homosexuality even where 'there is very little predisposition' will inevitably develop an inclination towards it.

However, these are but minor causes compared to the one that Hesnard feels is the most common cause: a dysfunctional relationship between mother and son:

> *Most of my patients, at an early age, were subject to the emotional influences of their mother, or of a rather masculine woman … who determined the law in the home. Occasionally their mother was very prudish or affected a supreme scorn towards questions of sex and love … the father being entirely out of the picture or forced into the background … this influence resulted in the child's acquiring a deep but apprehensive devotion to his mother.*

Hesnard goes on to explain that these boys then banish all thoughts of women being sexual or available as it conflicts with their idolisation of their mother, and so turn to homosexual experiences 'unworthy of their apparent virility'; Hesnard is not the only one to have favoured this line of enquiry.

It is no surprise that until very recent years, parents and especially mothers 'blamed' themselves for their son's homosexuality, wondering what they had done wrong either during pregnancy or as parents to cause this 'trait' in their beloved boy. The answer is as we now know, nothing – people are what they are, but in the confusing and often distressing process of getting to that realisation, untold damage was done to people with same-sex desires and indeed their families and familial relationships with these strange early 'explanations'. Hesnard also sees any form of

112

community spirit amongst homosexuals in a negative light, claiming that any mutual support, specific venues or recognition is a form of protest to show they are not different; the idea that at the time, homosexuals came together because they felt positively excluded by society does not seem to occur to him.

Hesnard is somewhat less positive in his pronouncements when it comes to 'cures' for homosexuals. He suggests that a cure which encourages a homosexual man to start a family is not a good idea and can only result in an unhappy home for the two partners, particularly when 'the seriousness of the *illness* [author's italics] does not appear until after the birth of the children.' He warns other therapists of the sensual attraction the homosexual will certainly feel towards his therapist (another reinforcement of the notion that all homosexuals seek sexual partners indiscriminately, which has no foundation in fact) and the patient will try to prolong therapy in order to keep seeing the doctor. Hesnard suggests that the therapist must be aware of this and stick to his plan to 'enoble and console' his client with spiritual development and 'sexual mastery through chastity', thus making the hapless pervert a boon to society in the end.

The last chapter in Hesnard's book is devoted to 'feminine homosexuality'. Here, we are told that all women are latently homosexual but that 'virtuous' women will resist this urge and confine themselves to passionate non-sexual friendships with other women instead. The idea that females are more likely to be bisexual is one that prevails to the present day, and may well be a throwback to the nineteenth-century acceptance of close female bonds as being harmless and to be tolerated, so long as they remain an accessory to a heterosexual marriage. Those women weak enough to succumb to their 'perverted' feelings are likely to be attracted to an opposite, in other words he sticks to the view of the Victorian sexologists that a masculine woman will always take as a lover a very feminine one. Hesnard blithely states that lesbians are generally manhaters (an accusation often wrongly thrown at the feminists later in the century, whether lesbian or not). Once again, we find the poor mothers of the lesbians getting the blame for their daughter's perversion; a baffling explanation includes a small girl confusing her erotic feelings for her mother with a fascination with her digestive system and her 'excretory organs' as he puts it, and feeling deeply possessive of her mother at the same time; one can't help feeling that, in scratching around

113

for an explanation for lesbianism that is different to the reasons for male homosexuality, Hesnard has got himself equally confused.

In order to give his book credibility, Hesnard also includes a section on examples of homosexuality in history and a brief description of earlier studies of the subject, and indeed, he was a respected therapist in his native France and beyond, as the American edition of his book illustrates – it was worth the publisher's expense to get the book translated into English. Of course, the vast majority of homosexuals, both male and female, would never even have heard of this man, but they would have felt his influence and that of others like him if they went to a doctor for help because this is exactly the sort of advice that was given to trainee psychologists at the time – homosexuals are sick; they have unique characteristics both physically and mentally; there is a strong link with neurosis; the problem started in their childhood; and they are hard to cure. Parents would end up being told by therapists and their homosexual children that apparently, they were to blame for this 'illness'; they too would then wholeheartedly want to 'cure' their child and may pressurise them into early marriages or aversion therapy. This overwhelming feeling of guilt is also felt by the child – guilt that their homosexuality has upset their parents – and so the cycle went on. Even decades later, this sort of misinformation was damaging family relationships. Lynn was a vivacious 14-year-old when she brought two homosexual friends back to the family home for tea. She already knew that she had feelings for other girls, and her two male friends understood and accepted her; she could talk to them freely without fear of bullying or other repercussions. The two teenage boys made no secret of their sexuality and came across as highly 'camp'. Lynn's mother met them in the hallway of the house, took one look at the boys and hissed to Lynn, 'In the kitchen. Now!'

Once out of earshot of the boys, her mother whispered aggressively 'Get rid of THEM. How dare you bring people *like that* to this house! What will the neighbours think?' Despite Lynn's futile protests, her mother was adamant. 'Get rid of them! I've a good mind to have you off to the doctor's for this in the morning!' Lynn had to go and tell her friends to leave – 'God, was Mum mad! It was highly embarrassing and the boys felt it too. And I thought "Well that's it, I can never tell her now."' The damage this incident did to Lynn was incalculable. She kept her sexuality a secret from her family, never able to tell her parents or her twin brother who she truly was. When her father accused the man living in the house opposite of being a 'pansy', a common derogatory word for a male homosexual at the time, she was even more reluctant to disclose her sexuality to anyone close to home. The threat of the doctor was enough to make her refuse to have any bloods taken when she was ill a few years later, as she feared her lesbianism would show up in the result – this may sound strange to the modern reader, but such was the mistrust of the medical profession that arose because of the fear of discovery and 'treatment'. Lynn had to move away from her native Merseyside simply in order to be herself and find happiness with a partner. In later life she said:

I could never, ever tell my Mum about myself, and I just feel she never really knew me because of that – and that makes me sad. I would have given anything to say her in those early days, "Mum, this is who I am." I knew how disappointed she would be in me, and that she would blame my being gay for all my past mistakes and breakdowns and I think she would have disowned me; she was a huge supporter of women being very feminine and men being the macho one. A big part of me was hidden from her. When I went to view her in the funeral director's just before her funeral, I told her then. It was a big sense of release. I hope that wherever she was, she heard me.

By this time Lynn had drifted apart from her brother, their careers taking them in completely different directions and to different parts of the country. At one point, Lynn's sister-in-law worked behind the bar of a gay bar in their home town; whether or not she had guessed her husband's sister was lesbian is not known, but she did try to gently encourage Lynn to visit the bar, saying what lovely people the clientele were. 'I couldn't go,' remembered Lynn. 'What if Mum had got to find out? I just couldn't risk that. So I told her I wasn't interested, which of course was a big lie.' Many years later, brother and sister briefly got back together. The brother said, 'If you not getting in touch is all about you being gay, I've known for years, since the days of Susan! It doesn't bother me if you are gay or not.' Susan was one of the rare girlfriends that Lynn had taken home, introducing her as a friend she worked with, 'But he never dobbed me in to Mum. That's loyalty for you.' The brother's response makes one wonder if the two siblings would have grown up closer if Lynn could have been honest about herself from the start, and this big secret had not been in the way.

Lynn's experience is far from unique. Many families throughout the first half of the twentieth century and beyond have whispered about, disciplined, and harangued their homosexual relatives, and even excluded them from the family unit; some, like Lynn, excluded themselves, because they felt it necessary to get away from their hometown and family in order to live a life true to themselves. By the 1930s, homosexuality had been taken from the clutches of being a crime against God and had been given to the doctors to cure. Not only were there the theories of mental disturbance, but some doctors also suggested a physical origin for homosexuality. In an answer to a Mass Observation Day Survey in 1937, respondent number 205 reported a conversation with a friend who had met a doctor researching the origins of homosexuality. The doctor stated that he thought it might be caused by 'pituitary disturbances'. The damage done to so many people by these early therapists and their theories – or even just the fear of them – is hard to excuse, or understand.

One young woman who was discovering her sexuality in the inter-wars years seems to have had an altogether better time of it. Born in 1914 to a poor working-class family in Blackburn, Barbara Bell had her first lesbian experience aged 14 and, in her mid-teens, even managed to persuade her parents to pay for what she describes in her autobiography as a 'mannish' suit made for her by a tailor. This suit, crafted in about 1931:

> ... was the first really mannish suit I had. Woollen material, air–force blue with a pinstripe. The skirt fitted over the hips, then very slightly flared. It had a beautiful jacket, padded shoulders ... [and was worn with] a navy-blue pork pie hat that went with the suit ... I felt a million dollars. It really did something for my ego. It made me feel strong and really butch.

However, while Barbara's family were proud of her smart new look, neighbours were making negative comments, although whether that was because her girlfriend, Trudi, was German and there was some latent hostility after the First World War, is impossible to say. Later on, to please her mother, Barbara had boyfriends but in her mind, it was entirely platonic and to keep the family happy: '... it was all an act to me, just an act. They only had to undo the buttons of my blouse once and they'd had it.'

116

Always restless and looking for adventure, Barbara joined the Metropolitan Police, encouraged by her father, and made the acquaintance of a number of other lesbian officers, and lived with one.

The Second World War and Beyond

The advent of war yet again in 1939 was a mixed blessing for most people. Rationing, the loneliness of loved ones being away at war or engaged in civilian war work far away from home, and of course the bereavement of so many whose family and friends were killed, became everyday occurrences. Despite all this, many people looked back in later years and saw the war as a revelatory experience, having given them the opportunity to be more adventurous in their relationships, and more honest about who they were – and whom they desired. This freedom was tempered by the knowledge that in fascist states such as Germany and Italy, the official line was that only wholesome male–female relationships were normal and acceptable, and eventually after the war it became apparent that homosexuals had been incarcerated in concentration camps along with other groups persecuted by the Nazi regime in Europe; the pink triangle was the mark worn by homosexuals in the camps, whilst known lesbians were made to prostitute themselves for camp officers and soldiers to effect a 'cure' for their lesbianism.

Thankfully, British homosexuals suffered nothing like that level of cruelty in their own country, but the law was still vigorously applied.

In 1942, the writer J. R. Ackerley came across an upsetting trial in the Welsh town of Abergavenny. Twenty men were arrested and tried for homosexual behaviour; as the proceedings unfolded, one 19-year-old man committed suicide, and another had a stroke but was still made to stand trial in his disabled state. Their sentences ranged from a year to twelve years in prison. Outraged, Ackerley wrote to the *Spectator* to demand more compassion, but his words went unheeded. This was wartime, and it was almost as if these men had committed a breach of discipline and must be made an example of.

Meanwhile, many homosexual entertainers did their part by entertaining the troops. Ivor Novello, who had just been released from a month's prison sentence for 'fiddling' petrol coupons (there was a rumour that he was also being punished for something more personal too) and his beloved partner Bobby Andrews travelled to France and Belgium under the auspices of ENSA (Entertainments National Service Association). There they performed favourite songs for the servicemen and women, and Ivor found that his new song, *We'll Gather Lilacs* was so popular that he decided to put it in his next show, *Perchance to Dream*.

Not everybody seemed to relish the new freedoms, however. In 1942, Mrs Innes Margaret Kerr was awarded damages of £300 in the High Court against Adelaide Mary Lady John Kennedy, who had referred to Kerr as a lesbian. The case was brought under the 1891 Slander of Women Act which allowed a prosecution if the chastity of a woman had been called into disrepute. The defendant's lawyers claimed the act could not be used as grounds for bringing the case, as the men who drafted it in 1891 would not have known about lesbianism and therefore it was not part of the legislation. The judge was not so sure – as the 'phenomenon' of lesbianism had been known for 2,500 years, he thought they would most certainly have heard of it and indeed: 'To assume this to be the case one must assume that they had little or no knowledge of the ancient world', a fair point as the upper-class and well-educated men of government would certainly have had a classical education. In her own defence, Lady Kennedy claimed she had never even heard the word 'lesbian', and her defence suggested that the word itself did not impute chastity; however, Mr Justice Asquith thought differently, and said that it did, hence the substantial damages, adding that the accusation of lesbianism was in fact more damaging than being accused of fornication or adultery. His 'reserved' judgement as the *Gloucestershire Echo* (20 February 1942) put it included a musing about the back story to the incident: 'There is a certain mystery about the motive and actions of more than one of the protagonists. One could speculate indefinitely on why the action was brought and fought.'

Barbara Bell found the war a liberating time. She had taken to wearing the characteristic ring on the little finger of her left hand, a discreet sign to other lesbians that they both belonged to the 'sisterhood':

> *If you were a lesbian, you wore a signet ring bigger and bolder and better than your next friend's ring.* [Speaking of women joining armed services in the war] *It was a bit difficult in the war years when so many were in uniform … they all looked like lesbians and it wasn't so easily defined but when you saw the little finger ring you knew. If you were fixed up with somebody you'd also wear a wedding ring, third finger, left hand.*

CHAPTER THREE

Barbara also found that it was much more acceptable during these years to wear trousers on an everyday basis, as so many women had to wear them for work.

At the end of the war, many people had to return to families and spouses, knowing that their lives had been irrevocably changed. This applied to many people regardless of who they were attracted to – the challenges and freedoms of the war had changed some individuals beyond the recognition of their families, colleagues and spouses. Many married people had had affairs, and yet were expected to go back to their homes as if nothing had happened and pick up their old life, with that secret inside them. Hundreds of married women were 'caught out' and had illegitimate babies, children that then had to be put up for adoption because it was so obvious they were literally 'little strangers'. Some of those close bonds, affairs or deep relationships would have been with someone of the same gender. It was impossible to fit in to the old life again, and frictions inevitably occurred. The divorce rate went from 8,254 in 1939 to 15, 634 in 1945, but by 1947 when the majority of servicemen and women had returned home from the war, it had risen to a dramatic 60,254. At the same time as the government was striving to rebuild Britain after the war, some family units were collapsing, and the message of the wartime romance *Brief Encounter* (1945), a film based on Noel Coward's 1936 play *Still Life,* in which a middle-class man and woman 'almost' have an affair but, with admirable restraint, end the liaison despite the heartache it caused – was clearly not to everyone's taste.

Some divorces, on the surface, seemed to have little to do with the war and were more about outright passion. The *Nottingham Evening Post* of 29 April 1949 reported a divorce case in which the third party was a female lover – of the wife. The third party, who was not named in the report, was in the habit of dressing as a man (as the judge put it) and had exercised a 'ghastly and baleful' influence on Winifred Tillson of Derbyshire, so much so that the married woman left her husband and moved to London to be with her lover. Her husband, Thomas, and the rest of the family tried to persuade Winifred to return home, which she did, and then the lover sent her a telegram saying she would end her life if Winifred did not return to her. It would appear that the two women were reunited and at some point after that, Mr Tillson began divorce proceedings. Judge Willes, in the divorce court, expressed the following opinion: 'I am quite satisfied that the actions and conduct of this curious woman –

a most baleful influence for evil on the wife – persuaded the wife to leave her husband and to live with her in London.' A decree nisi was granted to end the ten-year marriage and the judge expressed his deepest sympathy for the now ex-husband, surmising that but for this bad influence, the marital split would never have happened. Former Lord Chief Justice Goddard took a similarly negative view of homosexuals in his maiden speech in the House of Lords in April 1948, reaffirming that if homosexuals could not be reformed, then they must be punished.

It was also now the turn of the government to stick to their promise of making a better life for all their citizens, a promise that was not kept after the First World War. One of the key figures in obtaining benefits for mothers with children was Eleanor Rathbone (1872–1946), daughter of the Liberal MP for Liverpool, William Rathbone, who also went on to represent as an independent from 1929 onwards. Her campaigning credentials were impeccable – initially a social worker in Liverpool, she was to play an important role in the women's suffrage movement, but her life's work was a campaign for family allowances and the betterment of conditions for women both in Britain and in India. In 1940, as the debate over what sort of society Britain should be after the war ended, Eleanor published 'The Case for Family Allowances' and after more parliamentary argument, a bill was finally introduced to give mothers of young children a small allowance. Quietly in the background, throughout all these campaigns, was the woman who shared Eleanor's life, Elizabeth Macadam. They had met in the early years of the twentieth century and remained together until Eleanor's death in 1946, living a private life as mundane and happy as any other couple with their pet cat and their motor touring holidays.

Eleanor and her partner Elizabeth, when away from the public eye, seemed to have lived a life of quiet domestic contentment. However, other women needed desperately to find some way of meeting and socialising with women like themselves. The Gateways Club in London opened in the 1930s and was popular with bohemians and artists, but it was only after the war that it started to generate a more lesbian clientele and was almost exclusively lesbian by the 1950s. Membership was relatively reasonable in price (it was a private club) and as the venue was only small it was extremely crowded. Gina was the proprietor and initially ran the club with her husband, but later shared the task with her lover, a woman known as Smithy. Other venues where lesbians felt safe to gather in London were the Raven and the Robin Hood public houses.

CHAPTER THREE

In 1951, Ivor Novello, still accompanied by his devoted partner Bobby, was working as hard as ever. However, signs of ill health were starting to show and he collapsed at home, suffering from a coronary thrombosis. In the early hours of 6 March, with Bobby by his side, he passed away. The public was devastated. The man who had given them their iconic song in the First World War, and buoyed them with glamorous musicals through the depression and the next war, was gone, and they deeply mourned his passing. Thousands of people watched his final journey to his funeral at Golders Green Crematorium, a service that was broadcast live. Nowhere in the press, or anywhere else, was the fact that Bobby was at his companion's side to the end recorded or commented on. One of the most significant relationships of Ivor's life was banished to obscurity, and not even his status as a beloved public figure could save it from that. However, if one reads the biography of Novello that came out in 1951, for those who knew how to look for the clues, the relationship is there in the book, carefully coded of course, because Bobby was far too important for the author, W McQueen-Pope, to leave out completely. The author sings Bobby's praises as a devoted friend, advisor and confidante, and has included some charming photographs of the two men together, and yet if he relates that the two men go away or spend time together, he is always at pains to state that there was a female friend present too – presumably to deflect speculation about Ivor. The reader learns that Bobby had introduced Ivor to the work of American homosexual poet Walt Whitman, a writer much admired by many men before them including Oscar Wilde, and Ivor was so taken with one of the poems (*The Tan Faced Prairie Boy*) that he set it to music; contemporary readers may well have known that Whitman was regarded as a gifted writer of poetry with homosexual themes. It could be said that it is admirable that the author of this biography, published so soon after Novello's death, was fond enough of his friend to want to protect him from unkind gossip and damage to his posthumous reputation – and of course Bobby survived his partner, so if exposed to scrutiny he may have come to the attention of the police, which would have been deeply distressing on top of his bereavement. One cannot always see shame and embarrassment in what those around a homosexual did by way of concealment, and this book may well be a good example of that; perhaps such concealment may have even been an act of platonic, protective love.

A need to be covert may well have influenced the growth of friendly bars, coffee houses and private clubs that began to emerge after 1945.

Major cities such as Manchester and London and resorts such as Brighton and Blackpool all had venues where people in the know could gather in relative safety (compared to the dangers of 'cruising' in public spaces). Some public houses and bars hosted homosexual nights or even became almost exclusively homosexual in their clientele. The Union pub in central Manchester, located by the canal in an area best known for prostitution, was a popular venue and still is today, although now it is at the heart of a thriving gay 'Village'. To many men and women, these places were a revelation, and some had never seen so many fellow homosexuals in one place before. In some cases it was a first introduction to cultural manifestations such as 'butch' and 'femme' women, or cross-dressing men. Such venues played their part in allowing people to be themselves, look for partners or lovers, and move towards an acceptance of who they were in a world where isolation was still the norm.

In 1948 and 1953, two important reports were published by American researcher Alfred Kinsey which began the challenge to the notion that homosexuality was an illness. Having interviewed over 10,000 white Americans across the country, his findings were striking. Anything up to half of the males interviewed stated they had had homosexual experiences, and more than a quarter of women had felt attraction to another female and a significant number of those reported long term same-sex relationships lasting years rather than weeks. Kinsey concluded that it was impossible to segregate homosexuals into their own human 'ghetto' when it was clear that all humans were on a scale of sexuality and that approximately ten per cent of the population was homosexual. He replaced the 'traditional' triad of sexuality with a seven-point sliding scale from exclusively homosexual to completely heterosexual, a dramatic move which added complexity to the spectrum of accepted sexualities and must have made many people think again about their own place on this new scale. It was his conclusion also that homosexuals were to be found in every walk of life, and every strata of society; the theories of a past age that same-sex attraction was either a low-class phenomenon or a high-brow one (depending on when you lived), but never universal, was now debunked and consigned to the history books. Whilst the vast majority of people of any sexuality would not read this report, and most would not hear of it except in tap room banter or newspaper reports, it was to influence their doctors, psychologists and psychiatrists in the long term. In another outspoken gesture, artist John Minton (1917–1957) wrote a strong letter to the *Listener* magazine of 12 January 1950, in which Minton took issue with the derogatory tone that was used against Oscar Wilde (poor Oscar, still being attacked all those years later!) in a newly published book. Minton pointed out the great contribution made by homosexuals to society and pleaded for a 'saner and more comprehensive attitude towards the homosexual in society'.

The 'Witch Hunt' of Homosexual Men

In 1952, Britain was still heavily influenced by their wartime ally, the United States, which by now was undergoing the paranoia of the McCarthy witch hunts, seeking out communists in particular but also homosexuals who, as usual, were being lumped in with the left wing as a subversive threat. In 1952, under the influence of American politics and prejudices, arrests of homosexual men in Britain rose sharply from 956 in 1938, to 3,757. The Home Secretary, Sir David Maxwell Fyfe, told the House of Commons that homosexuals were 'proselytisers' and that they would receive no quarter from him. Sir John Nott-Bower became the new Commissioner of Police at Scotland Yard in 1953. It is thought that he too was influenced to conduct his crackdown on homosexual activity after being persuaded of the successes of the McCarthy 'witch hunts' and armed with draconian laws and the backing of a moralistic media and public, he set about his task with an enthusiasm that bordered on the fanatical. In the same year, Labour Member of Parliament William Field was arrested in Piccadilly Circus on a charge of importuning men for an immoral purpose. Naturally, he lost his job. Bigger names were to fall; revered actor Sir John Gielgud was arrested in a public toilet on a charge of 'importuning for immoral purposes', was fined £10 by a magistrate, and had to suffer vicious attacks in the press who called for his knighthood to be stripped from him. Thankfully the theatre-going public was somewhat more understanding, and gave Gielgud a standing ovation the next time he walked on to a stage after his conviction, so the establishment's attempts to use public figures as an example to others did not always have the desired effect. Many men fell victim to the well established police tactic of using a good looking officer in civilian clothes as a 'bait' – he would approach a man suspected to be cottaging and speak to him in a friendly way; they might then go for a drink together and once the officer felt he had sufficient evidence to make an arrest, he revealed his true identity. 1953 was also the year that the nonplussed citizens of middle-England heard the word 'homosexual' coming out of their radio sets for the first time, spoken by Dr Jacob Bronowski on the programme *Behind the News*. In 1954, Lord Montagu was arrested along with two friends – Michael Pitt-Rivers, and Peter Wildeblood (a *Daily Mail* journalist) on charges of improper behaviour with two airmen two years previously. All three men were found guilty and sent to prison. At this time, men had to be especially careful in their relationships, casual or otherwise. It was certainly not the done thing to keep a record of contact details for friends and lovers, or to write or keep love letters or a diary, all of which could fall into the hands of the Police, or perhaps worse still, a blackmailer. One would avoid giving one's real name if possible, and never take a stranger home (because then of course they would know an address). If a man was arrested and had been careless – or sentimental – enough to keep contact details, all his contacts would then be arrested and questioned separately, sometimes being told that their friends had confessed to gross indecency even when this was not the case; feeling cornered, some men would confess, believing that they had already been betrayed. Men who had been arrested could be humiliated by police, verbally abused and bullied, and some were arrested multiple times, partly because they were known to the police and had become part of the file of 'usual suspects'. Michael James, speaking to Alkarim Jivani, the author of *It's Not Unusual*, described the constant fear of arrest:

> *I felt dirty, I felt they had sort of disfigured me – I really did feel as if they had torn my face away and ... [I had] all these gangling nerve ends ... I was terrified to go out ... even just to the shop. I was terrified that I was going to be picked up again by another police car, that they were after me.*

Some men who had fallen in love with their life partner and set up home with them were careful not to have any double beds at home in case the police came in to their house and saw them, drawing an obvious conclusion. Thus men who loved devotedly and loyally, were good citizens in every other way other than their sexuality (according to the law) were denied the simple joy of sharing a bed with their life partner and waking up in the morning next to them without fear of institutionalised bullying. This may be where a common family history anecdote comes from – that an uncle,

CHAPTER THREE

cousin or brother did share their house with a 'friend' for many years, 'but there was nothing in it, they had separate bedrooms/beds'. Having separate sleeping arrangements may not have been a choice, but an imposition by a society that was prejudiced against them, and not only would they not want to end up in court, they would not want to humiliate their family either, especially if there was a degree of acceptance of their relationship within that family. Of course, human beings can be infinitely resourceful, and it was not unknown for male partners to sometimes share a bed but to also make sure that both bedrooms looked regularly inhabited, with bedclothes that looked used, the standard clutter of a bedroom in each one with hair brushes, full wardrobes and so on. Even though this may sound like an amusing game, it was a response to the fear of being 'caught'.

Also in 1954, pioneering computer scientist Alan Turing (born 1912) was found dead at his home. Turing was the expert who cracked the 'Enigma Code', which gave the Allied forces such an advantage in the Second World War. He was homosexual, and in 1951 had begun an affair with a young man named Arnold Murray, which soon petered out. Soon after, his flat was burgled by Murray and foolishly, on being questioned, Turing admitted to the investigating police officers that he and Murray had been lovers. In other words, he guilelessly revealed he had broken the law. In February 1952, Turing and Murray were arrested on a charge of gross indecency. Turing was a professor at Manchester University and his colleagues went along to the courtroom to testify on his behalf; Murray received a conditional discharge but Turing was put on probation, so long as he agreed to go through a new treatment called 'organo-therapy' – designed to repress or eliminate his desire for men. Turing was to have female hormones injected into him for a year; he complied, but did not like the fact that it made his breasts grow, although he managed to make wry jokes about it to friends all the same. His career suffered, maybe because of the upsetting disruption he had, but also because he was now seen as a threat to security; the fine mind that had helped shorten the war was now seen as vulnerable to indiscreet pillow talk. As a homosexual, what was seen as an innate unreliability was to impact on the work he lived for, although the University of Manchester stayed loyal to him, allowing him to take up a position especially created for him after his probation ended.

However, on 8 June 1954, the unthinkable happened. Alan Turing's housekeeper found the cryptographer dead in his bed at his home

'Hollymeade' in Wilmslow, Cheshire, apparently the victim of cyanide poisoning. Close by was a part-eaten apple. Had Turing laced his apple with the poison and eaten it? Had one of the finest minds of the twentieth century, the man whose skill had helped shorten the war and yet who was still preyed upon by the establishment because of his sexuality, fallen victim to the humiliation, degradation and stigma of loving the wrong gender? This was twelve years before homosexuality between two men over the age of twenty-one was finally decriminalised. The coroner had no doubt about what had happened and saw the death unequivocally as suicide: 'I am forced to the conclusion that this was a deliberate act. In *a man of his type*, one never knows what his mental processes are going to do next.'

What did the coroner mean by 'a man of his type'? He could have been referring to the eccentric professor type, or Turing's huge intellectual talent, or someone who was widely known in his own academic sphere even if not always to the wider public, but this is unlikely. It is reasonable to conclude that the inquest took the view that Turing's homosexuality had surely been his downfall and even caused him to commit suicide by eating an apple he had laced with cyanide; yet the apple was not analysed for cyanide and the autopsy results seemed to suggest he may have died from inhalation of cyanide fumes from his home laboratory, rather than it being a deliberate act.

As the inquest records were destroyed as a matter of routine – all family historians will know that this frustrating procedure occurs on a regular basis – a thorough examination of the evidence is not now possible; but there is enough documentation left to dispute the conclusion of suicide and indeed to suggest that Turing's death was a tragic accident that robbed the nation of a brilliant mind and great character. This is not to belittle the impact of his homosexuality on his life, of course. Like thousands of other men of his generation, Turing found himself the wrong side of the law of the nation he had endeavoured to protect less than ten years before, and this blatant lack of gratitude towards a man who did so much for his country was partly what led to a public campaign, to request a royal pardon for Turing under the Royal Prerogative of Mercy. Interest in, and sympathy for, Turing had accelerated since 2012 when his achievements in the war at Bletchley Park, the government's codebreaking headquarters were finally revealed in detail. The pardon was granted on 24 December 2013; Chris Grayling, the Justice Secretary at that time, said: 'A pardon from the Queen is a fitting tribute to an exceptional man'. In October 2016, and after another long campaign which was supported by

Turing's surviving family, the right to posthumous pardon for all men convicted under the same law as Turing was won; it can only be awarded posthumously however, and at the time of writing, the arrangements for those men still living to apply for a pardon have yet to be finalised.

It is impossible to say whether or not the doctors who 'treated' Alan Turing's homosexuality with hormones really thought it would 'cure' him, or not. However, apparent cures were still the fashion at the time, and they included aversion therapy. This took the form of using emetics to make the person vomit on being shown photographs of men, or if that did not work, electro-convulsive shock therapy was used in the same way. Horrifying tales of other countries such as Germany using lobotomies as a cure circulated, but it was a remedy that did not find favour in Britain. It is a sad fact that men and women were both encouraged to undertake these 'cures', which persuaded them at the time of a number of assumptions: firstly that homosexuality was temporary and that as an illness or disorder, it could be cured and secondly, that if it was a moral disorder, or the result of some fundamental weakness of will in the person, that it could and should be resisted if one wanted a 'normal' life. Bearing in the mind the awe in which many people, especially from poor or working-class backgrounds, held their doctors, it is little wonder that they put the blame on themselves for all the 'trouble' they were causing and meekly went along with the 'treatments'. Walter Braun described this treatment in his book *Lesbian Love,* a treatment he says is based on Pavlov's theory of conditioned reflex:

> *Lesbians who want to make use of this treatment are shown into a dark room. Soft music is heard and pictures of handsome naked men are projected on a screen. Then very unpleasant noises are heard and on the screen appear pictures of females. Every picture of women that is projected is accompanied by a palpable and extremely unpleasant electric shock that is administered to the patient. The inventors of the treatment claim they were able to cure many homosexuals in this way.*

As more and more men of all types of build and personality began to fall foul of the law, it was increasingly clear that any stereotype of a homosexual man was limiting in the extreme. Menlove Edwards (1910–1958) was a strong, athletic man, a gifted climber and one of the great rock climbers of his times. Armed with his degree in medicine from Liverpool University, he decided to specialise in what we would now refer to as 'mental health issues' and set up clinic as a psychiatrist. This gifted man also wrote poetry and in 1935 he gave a sermon at Stokesay church in Shropshire (his brother was the vicar there), calling for understanding of homosexuals and stating his view that homosexuality and Christianity could be reconciled. When the Second World War started, Menlove registered as a conscientious objector, so he also had the courage of his convictions, but as he was not allowed to practise as a result, he spent the war in Wales working on his research. Menlove was not a man who fitted into the caricature of a limp wristed, foppish male who only had frivolous thoughts and lived only to have a 'good time'. Here was a serious professional man, strong and competent, who just happened to fall in love with other men, who did not cruise the streets looking for casual sex so far as we know, but had meaningful relationships instead. At all times in history, it is a mistake to assume that all people within a group whom are collectively given a certain label, can be seen as the same, and homosexual men and women are equally as diverse as any other demographic group.

However, opinion seemed to be shifting. Perhaps because they feared for their own homosexual friends and relatives, people were finding the witch hunt of men who loved men was just too much. The airmen who testified against the Montagu trio were booed; serious newspapers started suggesting that public opinion was more enlightened than the law. For the first time, the House of Lords held a debate into the issue of homosexuality. Finally, in 1954, Sir John Wolfenden QC was asked to spearhead an enquiry into the matter, and a committee was appointed on 4 August. By the time the committee was set up, all major legislation dealing with male homosexuality had been lumped in with acts of parliament which attempted to control female prostitution – The Criminal Law Amendment acts (1885 and 1912), and the Vagrancy Act (1898), and it is worth remembering the full title of the Committee: The Departmental Committee on Homosexual Offences and Prostitution, as its remit went beyond just that of studying the law and homosexuality. The fifteen strong committee, which included judges, MPs, doctors, lawyers, clergymen, and the female chair of the Scottish Association of Girls' Clubs, took two years to deliberate the subject of the law and homosexual men. Two hundred people gave evidence to the committee, and it met sixty-two times; E. M. Forster finally stuck his head above the parapet and wrote an article for the *New Statesman* in 1955 arguing for reform of the law. The committee discovered that half of all blackmail cases reported to the police from 1950–53 involved homosexual men, which shows just how frightened men were of blackmail if they preferred the scrutiny of the police to blackmail.

Forster would have been pleased with the conclusion of the committee, which recommended that: 'Homosexual behaviour between consenting adults in private should no longer be a criminal offence'. It also recommended that the age of consent for male homosexual relations be fixed at 21 years, which would put it in line with France. Unfortunately this was still out of line with everyone else, as heterosexuals and lesbians could legally have a sexual relationship from the age of 16. This was a big news story, but not everyone was in favour of reform. Only a minority of people questioned by Gallop for a poll wanted decriminalisation, and the *Express*, whose Sunday edition had begun the campaign against Radclyffe Hall's *The Well of Loneliness*, was highly critical. MPs debated the report in November 1957, with the usual objections being made as they had been for many years, to any relaxation of the law. The majority of Liberal and Labour MPs supported a liberalisation of the law, but without an overall majority, not much could be done, and 'Rab' Butler, the Tory Home Secretary, was in no hurry to help. This ground breaking report and its recommendations, so brave for the times, was to languish on the shelf until a more vigorous and open campaign to change the law was eventually heard.

In 1955, following his release from prison after a sentence for homosexual offences, Peter Wildeblood wrote *Against the Law*. In it he demanded acceptance for more conventional homosexuals like himself but did not make the same appeal on behalf of less masculine homosexuals – 'The pathetically flamboyant pansy with the flapping wrists ... the effeminate creatures who love to make an exhibition of themselves'. This lack of unity can be forgiven if one considers the pressure homosexual men were under at this time; any association with men who were so openly, gloriously themselves was dangerous and could lead to arrest and imprisonment. If one could be seen and accepted as respectable, law abiding and just plain ordinary in every way except for one's romantic preferences, life could be so much easier. Wildeblood was not the only person who focussed on stereotypes. Therapist Walter Braun wrote:

> *Male homosexuals have a preference for certain professions. The feminine type ... likes to work as a fashion designer,*

a window dresser, a ballet dancer or hairdresser. The masculine type sometimes is sailor, truck driver or boxer.

Ordinary lesbians and homosexuals knew differently; they knew they were simply people in the widest possible spectrum of jobs – nurses, soldiers, teachers, priests, builders, lawyers, police officers, home makers, labourers – who simply wanted to get on with their lives and set up home with a special person like their heterosexual friends and family did. Far from wanting to be defined by their choice of partner, they wanted, like everyone else, to be defined by the calibre of person they were. It would take several more decades to approach that level of acceptance in society.

Public figures with high popularity ratings and reputations to protect were guarded in their support for reform, in public at any rate. In his diary for 10 November 1955, Noel Coward wrote passionately and at length against the current laws regarding homosexuality: 'Emotional, uninformed prejudice can still send men to prison and ruin their lives for a crime that in the eyes of any intelligent human being is not a crime at all … to attempt by law to eliminate it is as foolish as to try to eliminate hair colouring and skin pigmentation.' One wonders what reaction his very long plea for acceptance, of which this is a tiny part, would have caused had he sent it to a newspaper at the time. Women's lives contracted back to the home yet again, their services no longer required after the war; the fashion retailers gladly supplied the ultra-feminine styles of the New Look, a reaction to fashion austerity of the war years. Gone were the androgynous styles that characterised the aftermath of the First World War and which, to an extent, allowed some lesbians to express their masculinity under a cover of being 'fashionable'. Women's magazines featured housewives in brightly coloured aprons serving up home cooked meals to their very masculine husbands and rosy-cheeked children; their problem pages continued to sternly advise any female who wrote to them because they were struggling with their same-sex feelings that it was simply a crush and they should grow up quickly and find a nice young gentleman or pull themselves together and concentrate on their husband. Even though lesbian relationships were in no way against the law, they were still frowned upon and not spoken of, and for many in the provinces, especially in rural settings, it was nearly impossible to meet other lesbians. The first lesbian magazine with a decent circulation – *Arena Three* – did not begin until 1964. As late as 1966, Walter Braun, although a sympathetic writer in favour of a pragmatic acceptance of the fact of homosexuality, relates a case study of a woman who, with the aid of his therapy, had 'successfully' repressed her lesbianism in order to get married and have a child, and stated she was very happy so long as she could continue to keep her same-sex desires under strict control. In the same year, Bryan Magee made the first of two television programmes about homosexuality and shortly afterwards collated his research into a book, *One in Twenty*. Even in the mid 1960s, Magee was baffled to find that there was still a misconception that lesbians were predatory and would 'seduce and corrupt people', even in the workplace (although it must be said that he was not entirely uncritical of the dynamics of a lesbian partnership, labelling it emotionally stifling). In 1956, The Sexual Offences Act became law and recognised the crime of sexual assault between women, a strange form of acceptance by the government that lesbian relationships existed, a sign of equality of sorts, and of the fact that there was still confusion and prejudice in the oddest places.

In the same year, the Civil Service's Statement on the Findings of the Conference of Privy Councillors, mentioned homosexuality as a 'character defect' for the first time, which cannot have helped the confidence of what must have been hundreds of lesbian and homosexual civil servants.

There was clearly so much more to be done. In 1957, there was still a ban on theatre performances with overtly homosexual themes. The opportunities for homosexual men and women to meet freely at social venues without fear of being targeted were still very limited, in particular outside the larger cities. Thanks to a cultural regression after the end of the Second World War, many governments and societies became more conservative and indeed repressive, as the McCarthy witch hunts of 'communists' shows. Homosexuality became readily linked with communism, as if one was a prerequisite for the other, an absurd idea – the same spectrum of political ideology occurs in the homosexual community as in any other. The 'Swinging Sixties' and its cultural freedoms and legal liberalisations had not happened yet – groundbreaking movies such as *Victim* (1961) starring Dirk Bogarde, himself homosexual and playing a man who was being blackmailed because of his sexuality, had yet to happen. It is too easy to think that the Wolfenden Report was a watershed, but in fact it was only a step along the way.

Afterword

It is hoped that this narrative has opened up a new subject to the family and social history researcher, and put those of our ancestors who fell in love with someone of the same gender firmly in their family and societal setting. Looking back at the history of same-sex relationships, the same patterns emerge as can be seen today. There was, and is, the widest spectrum of relationships between people of the same gender. There were romantic friendships, passionate friendships, others that were passionately sexual, and yet others that were asexual, based on a deep love that knew no sexual or erotic element at all – each mirroring the huge variety of heterosexual relationships that can be found throughout history. In the twenty-first century, society accepts that people can be anywhere on a spectrum of sexuality and that they will hope for successful relationships just like everyone else. If this is so, then the same applies to people in the past, although of course they did not have the self-knowledge or the 'labels' to identify with, or the acceptance in society to be themselves. Despite this they struggled to love and live in their own unique ways. We can never know for most of them exactly how important a sexual element was in their relationships, or even if there was one; this lack of knowing means one cannot define a same-sex relationship exclusively with sexual parameters. To put it simply, perhaps it is time that we recognised the diversity of relationships in history and celebrated that above all, just as we do today.

Search Terms of use to Those Researching Same-Sex Relationships

(Of use when searching online or in archive catalogues)

GENERAL/BOTH GENDERS

Bisexual
Cross dressing
Deviant
Disorderly house
Drag
Homogenic
Homosexual, homosexuals
Intermediate sex
Inverts, Inversion (sexual)
Onanist, onanism
Same sex
Sexual minorities
Sexual transgression
Sexuality
Sexual orientation
Third sex
Transvestite
Unnatural acts
Unnatural offences
Urning

FOR MEN

Buggery
Catamite

Effeminatus
Ganymede
Gay
Greek Love
Gross indecency
Importuning
Indecency
Margery/ie
Men dressed as women
Obscenity
Poof/f
Queer, queers
Sodomy, sodomite
Soliciting
Street offences
Transvestism
Uranian

FOR WOMEN

Butch
Female husband
Femme
Flatting, the Flat(t)s
Frictrice
Hermaphrodite
Lesbian, lesbians
Passing women
Sapphist, sapphic
Tom, Tommy
Transvestism
Tribade
Women dressed as men

**FAMILY HISTORY AND OTHER ARCHIVAL SOURCES
(for example, any of the above terms plus …..)**

Census returns

APPENDIX I

Court Records
Divorce
Irregular marriages
Maps (venues, addresses etc)
Newspapers
Parish Registers
Personal papers (letters, diaries, address books, postcards, greetings cards etc)
Photographs (venues, addresses, public spaces, people)
Police and Prison records
Popular culture (theatrical ephemera, playbills, song/ballad sheets, broadsheets, chapbooks)
Same-sex marriages (parish registers)
Trade Directories (individuals, businesses, social venues)
Trade Ephemera (letterheads for venues, flyers, posters, etc)
Visual sources other than photographs (paintings, drawings, etchings, etc.)

Note – any of the above can also be refined by adding place names, dates, etc.

The Attenders at the Masked Ball, Hulme, Manchester, September 1880

(Format of information is as follows: Name, age, address, marital status, occupation, whether or not cross-dressing indicated by CD Yes or CD No, as far as is known)

Ainsworth Earnshaw, John, 25, 35 Alexandra Street, Lower Broughton, Salford, single, stonemason, CD No

Allse, Charles, 21, 1 Penny Lane Stockport, single, factory operative, CD No

Bingham, George, 36, 43 Penistone Road, Sheffield, single, metal worker, CD No

Broughton, George, 30, 62 Wakefield Road, Stalybridge, marital status not known, schoolmaster, CD Yes

Buckmaster, Alfred, 26, 4 Albion Place, Halliwell Lane, Cheetham, Manchester, single, clerk, CD No

Buxton, George, 26, 87 Port Street, marital status not known, fustian cutter, CD No

Cartwright, Jon, 25, 62 Wakefield Road, Stalybridge (note this is the same address as George Broughton), marital status not known, draper, CD No

Coore, John Henry, age not known, 110 Slater Street, Oldham Road, Manchester, single, shopkeeper, CD No

Dickinson, James, age not known, 5 Ivy Grove, Chapman Street, Hulme, marital status not known, waiter, CD No

Fox, Robert, 28, 73 Tamworth Street, Stretford Road, Hulme, single, jewellers assistant, CD No

APPENDIX II

Frudd, William, age not known, 62 Johnson Street, Sheffield, single, Carriage trimmer, CD No

Gorton, Arthur Henry, 22, 94 Regent Road, marital status not known, bookkeeper, CD No

Haslam, Isaac, 36, 53 South Street, Park Sheffield, single, shopkeeper, CD No

Holliday, John (also known as Nathan), 16, 7 Ruby Street, Boundary Lane, Manchester, single, plumber, CD Yes

Ingham, William, 31, 12 Weaste Lane, Eccles, single, butler, CD No

Jackson, James William, 19, of Oldham, single, a piecer, CD No

Jackson, William, 22, of Manchester, single, salesman, CD No

Jepson, James William, 19, 15 Ash Street, Oldham, single, piecer, CD No

Kirby, Richard, 30, 36 Godson Street, Oldham, married, clerk, CD No

Lomas, Arthur, 29, No 2 Court, 8 Allen Street, married, drawing master, CD Yes (noted as 'very convincing')

Lythgoe, James, 24, 12 Windsor Terrace, Windsor Bridge, single, clerk, CD No

Marloe, James, 19, 4 Gilbraltar Street, Lees, Oldham, single, carter, CD No

Mellor, James, 19, of Leeds, single, a carter, CD No

Monaghan, Thomas, 32, 37 Birch Street, Hulme, single, bill poster, CD No

Montrasser, Frederick, 21, address not known, single, waiter at Farbon's Restaurant, Cannon Street, Manchester, CD Yes

Oates, William, 28, 2 Little Camp Street, marital status not known, porter, CD Yes

Ogden, Abraham, 21, 77 Great Jackson Street, Hulme, single, baker, CD No

Parkinson, Ernest, 19, Victoria House, Spring Road, Bury, single, singer, CD No

Parry, Henry, 33, 6 Fern Court, Silver Street, Hulme, single, painter, CD No

Pickens, Edward, 25, 25 Marple Street, Chorlton Road, Hulme, single, bookbinder, CD Yes

Pitt, Thomas, 22, 102 Union Street, Ashton Under Lyne, single, draper, CD Yes

Powell, Edward, 23, 59 Woodhead Road, Sheffield, single, gilder, CD No

Price, John, 20, 5 Ogden Street, Bedford Street, Hulme, single, hawker, CD No

Rennie, William, 26, 14 Heywood Street, Oldham, single, mechanic, CD No

Richardson, Frederick, 28, 3 Dronfield Road, Sheffield, single, confectioner, CD No

Saxton, Nathaniel, 25, back of 23 Grove Street, Sheffield, single, waiter, CD No

Shawcross, Arthur, 48, 11 Elizabeth Street, West Gorton, single, mechanic, CD No

Shufflebottom, Abraham, 38, of Salford, Married, hawker, CD No

Southern, William, 27, 17 Sofia Street, Rochdale Road and Stand Avenue Cheetwood (Cheetham Hill, Manchester), single, chemist, CD No

Smith, Frank, 24, 13 Spittall Street, Oldham Road, Manchester, marital status not known, dancer, CD Yes

Speed, Charles, 45, 77 Monmouth Street, Sheffield, single, finisher, CD No

Towney, Charles, 37, of Miles Platting, married, dyer, CD No

Walker, Richard, 40, 31 Lower Chatham Street, Chorlton-upon-Medlock, Manchester, single, waiter, CD No

Warburton, James, 32, 10 Winford Street, Eccles New Road, single, waiter, CD No

Whitehead, Edward, 20, 11 Huntingdon Street, Oxford Road, Manchester, single, bottle maker, CD No

Whiteman, Thomas, 18, 3 Sickle Street, Waterloo Street, Oldham, single, grocer, CD Yes

Whitworth, Thomas, 23, 8 Rodney Lane, marital status not known, silversmith, CD No

A Research Guide to Same-Sex Relationships

Be Flexible

This book has aimed to show the reader that the concept of same-sex relationships is much more nuanced than it would first appear. It follows that when researching this subject, or rather when trying to find out about the lives of those who were involved in a same-sex connection, again the researcher has to be on their toes to use every resource at their disposal to rebuild the picture of those lives. Some, such as a same-sex household comprising two people living together for economic or companionship reasons, may have had no thoughts that they should conceal anything about their lives, and they may be easier to track down in the records. However, if the household is built on a romantic or sexual relationship, the temptation is there to conceal facts that could lead the authorities to draw, not the wrong conclusion, but alas, the right one. So the first thing a researcher in this field needs to be is flexible, and to think laterally as circumstances dictate:

1. Use the expertise of local archivists if you are researching in a 'real' rather than online archive. They will be familiar with their indexing techniques and will know what words have been used as identifiers for anything relating to same-sex relationships, court cases, and so on. A list of words you may want to look for in catalogues is given in Appendix I. Also, archivists have more than likely been asked for such material before and could save you a lot of time by going straight to the items you need rather than you having to search.

2. Look around the subject. Why would a cross-dressing woman and her 'wife' live in a particular street or area? Are there indicators that it could have been a safe haven for them, and why? In a very poor area with much petty crime, it was in no one's interests to have the authorities poking around just because someone complained about the two women

living a few doors away, not so much honour amongst thieves as loyalty amongst the downtrodden. Putting people into the context of their time and place will help you understand them and their life choices. Finding out about the life of an academic at a provincial university in the middle of the twentieth century could give you insights into the work of Alan Turing, for instance; understanding where Harry Stokes chose to live may also reveal something about how she lived and thought.

3. Think laterally about names. This is always vital to any family historian but becomes even more important when it comes to those who have adopted a new 'persona', may have cross dressed, or were in some way apart from the conventions of family and naming. Author Radclyffe Hall much preferred her friends to call her John, but nowhere on her official records will you see this name, she is always listed by her full birth name of Marguerite Radclyffe Hall. However, look at any greetings cards or letters sent to her by her close circle and she will be addressed as John. Many people have family or pet names, but homosexuals may have had others still. Perhaps there is a story in the family that your great-great Aunt, who lived with her 'friend' for twenty years till one of them died, was known to her friends and close family as Tommy? Tommy was a word used for lesbians in the later nineteenth century. An in joke like this could be invaluable in building up a picture of that person's life, but do not hope for it to be her name on a census return, will, receipt or letterhead, or a civil registration certificate. Again, if someone has adopted the name of their 'spouse' (perhaps for the sake of conventionality, if one is a cross-dressing partner, and so on) then look for them under a combination of all or any of their names. Hyphenated names were less common in the age of available census returns compared to the later twentieth and early twenty-first century, but one surname may be listed as a middle name (don't assume which way round they will be!). As always, make lists of the possible names a person could be known by, and bear them in mind when searching records, ticking them off as you check them so you don't repeat the search and end up going round in circles.

Be Realistic

Family historians are only too well aware that when a relative or ancestor dies, the likelihood is that there will be the usual 'clear out'. The deceased's effects and papers must be put in order, the house emptied or sold, and the requirements of the will honoured. However, grieving relatives may also have another important task to do: the construction of the deceased person's legacy. Love letters, especially if they are in connection with a relationship that was extra marital, will be destroyed. Useful items such as documents giving past addresses, postcards, greetings cards and mementoes, diaries, and address books are all at risk. One family historian arrived at the home of her recently deceased, very elderly uncle to find her cousin in the back garden, piling all uncle's papers into a garden incinerator from which flames shot up like an upturned rocket. All uncle's family papers were gone forever, because the cousin, who was not a genealogist, saw all these items as so much rubbish and in her mind, was simply and helpfully making a start on clearing the house.

Imagine how much more sensitive many relatives and bereaved partners would feel if the deceased was a person with same-sex desires or relationships. Examples of reputations being posthumously 'sanitised' abound. After the death of author Radclyffe Hall in 1943, her 'spouse', Una Troubridge, kept her promise to Hall to destroy the unfinished manuscript of the latest novel. Una also tried hard, however, to obliterate any connection between Hall and her former mistress, Evgenia Souline. Una burned all the letters that Souline had sent to her lover, hoping to restore a pure image of her own long partnership with Hall. She very soon began writing her own account of Hall's life – she did not exclude Souline from it, but described her as a querulous hanger-on who threw Hall's goodwill back in her face and played with her emotions. It was all a fruitless exercise – Souline had kept all the letters Hall had sent her, and they have now been published, a passionate and detailed account of a doomed love affair that embroiled all three women in a destructive cycle of recrimination and anguish. There was no denying that Hall was lesbian – she had made a sort of career out of sacrificing herself to the cause of visibility – but what kind of lesbian she was could be manipulated.

The niece of American poet Emily Dickinson set to work after Dickinson's death to burn all the adoring letters that she had sent to the niece's mother, Susan Gilbert, as she did not want their close friendship to be revealed to the public at any point. Thankfully, some letters survived.

All this is a process of denial and the preservation of the family name and that of the deceased. The Lesbian History Group calls this process the 'normalising process'. It seems ridiculous to many researchers today that such lengths were gone to, to obliterate significant parts of a person's very being and who they were, but this denial also extended beyond family and partners to the media and historians and biographers. Such was the success of these destroyers of life records in some cases, that the sexuality of the deceased is blurred and it is then easier to 'normalise' it – which is undoubtedly what the destroyers (and sometimes the deceased) wanted.

Assumptions and Educated Guesswork

This book does not aim to create same-sex relationships where none existed. It aims to be a straightforward account of the lives of those who loved others of the same gender, and when family historians investigate ancestors who may or may not have loved someone of the same sex, they must not assume either. Do not add a same-sex household to your file of family history stories unless you have good reason to do so. Also, do not assume a sexual partnership unless you have reason to do so. This is extremely difficult, as within a heterosexual marriage we tend to assume that the children born into it are the product of a sexual relationship between the husband and wife (whether or not we *should* assume is a study that would make a book in its own right).

In addition, do not expect any ancestor who may have been homosexual to look a certain way. The likes of Oscar Wilde – affluent, well-educated, urbane, aesthetic – were unusual. Women who passed as male in order to make a better living for themselves and their 'wife' (and for many of them, we have no firm evidence that they would identify as transgendered today, so as historians we must not assume) were in the minority; most women who loved women wore clothes as decorative and elaborate as any heterosexual woman. They may have toned them down somewhat, but in many cases conventions were adhered to. Radclyffe Hall still had her beautiful, blonde, waist-length hair till her thirties, and although many photographs of her show her sporting a jacket, shirt and tie tailored in a masculine way, what they rarely show is that she almost always wore a skirt to match, not trousers. Pit brow girls at the Victorian coal mines in Lancashire wore trousers to work every day, but only a small proportion of them would have fallen in love with another woman. Richard Findlater, who wrote a biography of Lilian Baylis, the noted feminist, claimed she was not 'mannish and butch' enough to be lesbian, and 'was, in fact, for all her brusqueness and bossiness, a very feminine woman'. Do not fall into the derogatory trap of thinking a woman was 'too pretty' or feminine to be lesbian, and likewise, do not assume a woman is lesbian simply because she seems masculine, lived alone, or comes across as very independent for her generation. Gender is much more complex than that; never make assumptions on the basis of appearance.

142

Lies, Secrecy and Confidentiality

Making homosexuality illegal or immoral seems to most people in Britain today to be at least unfair and at worst, despicable. To force people to repress their sexuality – an aspect of their very being that they can do nothing about – and expect them to either enter into unsatisfactory marriages or remain alone apart from brief, secret flings all their adult lives is nothing short of cruel. However, the secrecy that was forced on homosexual men and women in the past is in fact a double-edged sword for the researcher. If there are laws to be transgressed, someone is bound to do just that, and that will lead to police records, possibly a trial or appearance at the magistrate's court, and almost certainly reports in the press both local and national. As we have seen, not just men but women also could be embroiled in a scandal that swept away their efforts at secrecy and put them in the glare of public attention.

However, the reverse side of this is the lack of records of a personal nature, the sorts of records that are not replicated in any official source. These might be destroyed before death, after death by a loved one, or simply never kept at all. If there is nothing of this nature in the family archive, a broader sweep must be undertaken. If you do think your ancestor socialised with other homosexuals, male or female, in a certain locality, you can at least find out about the venues they could have used, the networks that might have supported them, and possibly there will be oral history sources you can access that can give you an idea of what life was like for them.

Also, what about the photo of Aunty which has clearly been cut in half, and the family rumour is that Aunty's mother chopped it up because the missing half showed Aunty's long standing 'friend'? Many studio photos in the past, especially in the twentieth century, were bought in lots of half a dozen, so out there in the wider family may be whole copies of that photograph. Online networking with extended family may bring it to light, and those more distant relatives may have information about Aunty and her friend that was never spoken at home because it was – literally – too close to home; extended family may have been more willing to gossip about it, this might have been overheard by curious children, and those stories may now be accessible to you. (see the comments on safe networking in the resources section before you embark on a search like this). As always, of course, beware the assumptions about a person based on appearance or half-hearted rumour. In his diary entry for 19 March 1955, Noel Coward reflected wryly on what would be said about him after his death, having led so discreet a public life:

... the only thing that saddens me over my demise is that I shall not be here to read the nonsense that will be written about me and my works and my motives. There will be books proving conclusively that I was homosexual and books proving equally that I was not. There will be detailed and inaccurate analyses of my motives for writing this or that and of my character.

If a famous person thought that, think how much more difficult it is to build the life of an anonymous, ordinary member of a working-class or middle-class family!

SAMPLE RESEARCH PROJECT FOR A SAME SEX PROJECT

(taken from a real case, with names and location changed)

The Scenario

In 1938, a businessman is found guilty of two charges of gross indecency with male persons and sentenced to two years in prison. Two other charges have been dropped due to a lack of corroboration, so the sentence is reduced to nine months in prison. The man's name is Peter Holden and he lives in a city in West Yorkshire. How can we find out about him, and his life?

What Resources Can be Used?

Peter is an adult and has his own business. It is possible that he will be on the 1911 census, to which we have access. He will more than likely be young – even a child – and to find him in the context of his family will give insights into his social and economic status. He may even be on the 1901 census or the 1891 census. Later censuses are not available.

Business: As a businessman Peter may well have premises, these can be searched for in trade directories, on maps (Ordnance Survey and Goads fire insurance maps) and in visual archives (the shop front). There may be trade ephemera such as catalogues and letterheads. If it is a family business, his role in it may be harder to ascertain. He may have been a member of local trade associations and he more than likely has a telephone and can be traced in the directories for that. What might have happened to Peter's business whilst he was in prison? Family may have stepped in and kept it going, or they may have worked in it anyway. Alternatively, the business may have been sold – look for advertisements offering businesses for sale, or records of bankruptcy proceedings.

Addresses: He may well have two addresses, one for work and another home address. Electoral registers can also be checked to see if Peter moved house, especially after his release from prison. Again, did Peter have to sell his house if he owned one? Look for house sale advertisements. Check electoral registers to see if Peter lived alone, and if not, with whom. Any persons at that address who may have been his partner – male or female? After his release from prison, does he still live with them, or anyone else? It may help show if his friends and family stood by him or not. If you cannot find Peter after his release from prison, be liberal in your searches for his new address, as he may have decided to move to a new area, or he may have had to move because of the war. See also 1939 National Registration, below.

Legal: Peter will be in court and police records but the 100-year rule may apply to some of these, if not all. Newspaper reports may fill in the gaps about his trial and may even reveal if there were any other defendants named. Check to see if Peter appealed his sentence, and what happened to the appeal.

Lifestyle: What was it like for men and women seeking same-sex partners in the area Peter lived in? Where did they meet? Are there any records for this? Perhaps Peter was entrapped in a police 'sting', but that does not mean there were no meeting places there too. Local archives or specialist lesbian and gay archives may be able to help with information but do not expect lists of names or photographs showing Peter and his friends. There may be oral history recordings describing what life was like for homosexuals in Peter's home town that will help give a picture of what his life was like. If there are no records like this, take a broad sweep of local newspapers and see what comes up in the way of other cases, which might give background information.

Life events: was Peter married and did he have children? Check the civil registration indexes for life events connected with him. Was he ever divorced? Local courts or archives, depending on date, will have some records that you may have access to. If, tragically, Peter committed suicide, his death certificate will show this and you may be able to access coroner's records or at least newspaper reports.

Wills: as a businessman, Peter may have been able to keep going and been affluent enough to leave a will when he died. A copy should be available through the national index to wills copy service. This may show family and close friends and his whereabouts when he died.

War service: If old enough, Peter may have served in the First World War and his service records may have survived (although remember that survival rates for army records in particular are poor). It is possible he served in the Second World War in some capacity and even Home Guard records are now available to search online on a subscription based website.

Medical records: Did Peter go though aversion or other psychiatric therapy because of his sexuality or for any other reason? Records may survive but access will be limited within the 100-year rule. Check instead to find out what the medical policy was for the hospital services where he lived, to get an idea of what he may have endured.

1939 National Registration: you may have access to the entries showing Peter, depending on whether or not he is now deceased. As time goes by, more of this resource will become available but at present access is limited somewhat.

Information about Peter's sexuality: this will more than likely be limited to the newspaper reports of his trial. There may also be family stories about Peter amongst living relatives or others who knew him. See the advice about online networking, and proceed with caution.

Archival Resources that may help the general research of homosexuals 1700–1957:

1. *Census Enumerator's returns, 1841–1911*

   Invaluable resource which can be searched online via name, address, or other key words (not those describing homosexuals, of course). The usual caveats apply – beware of stated relationships such as a partner listed as a lodger or visitor, that would be to maintain an element of respectability. Be liberal with how you search regarding names, and if there are aliases, try all of them. Do not assume a homosexual was able to stay in the same place all the time especially after a brush with the law. Always endeavour to view the original document in digitised form, do not rely on transcriptions. If the person you are looking for is in the same place as their family, try plotting their addresses on a contemporary map as this will give you an idea of how close your subject lived to their family. This in turn may give an indication of whether or not they were still in touch.

Location: this will always be online in some format. See the list of websites for suggestions.

2. *Parish Registers*

Not just attempted same-sex marriages but the marriages of the countless homosexuals over the years who have married in a conventional way. Baptisms and burials for your subject and their family may also be listed.

Location: Many parish registers are now online but you will probably have to pay a subscription to a website to use them. Originals for the Anglican Church are usually held at the relevant county archive and will also be on microfilm/fiche. Rarely, they are kept at the church itself.

3. *Newspapers*

There are literally thousands of scanned, digital versions of old newspapers now online, which can be invaluable in following the fortunes of individuals, especially where they were unfortunate enough to find themselves in court. See the list of websites for online collections, most of which are either integrated into a major family history search website, or are 'stand-alone' websites. Most of these collections require a subscription to access them, but if your local library subscribes to a website such as Ancestry or Find My Past, you will have free access to the newspaper section through that if you have a valid library ticket. You will more than likely have to visit the library in person, it is rarely, if ever, a service offered via your home computer. If you have names and dates, use those to search for news stories, but the usual proviso of being flexible about spellings of names applies. Also, do not restrict your search to a specific newspaper. Of course the local newspaper will, or should, have good coverage, but the story may well have been syndicated to many other newspapers around the country, and each article may add details of interest. If you are not looking for a specific person but browsing for any news story relating to the subject, use the list of key words in Appendix I to help you find articles.

Bear in mind that newspapers are there to entertain as much as to inform, so make sure you verify facts where you can before adding them to your family history.

Newspapers and journals consulted for this book:

The Blackburn Standard
Chester Courant
Daily Herald
Daily Mail
Derby Daily Telegraph
Dundee Courier
The Gentleman's Magazine
Gloucestershire Echo
Kent Weekly Post or Canterbury Journal
Lancaster Gazette
Liverpool Mercury
London Evening Standard
Manchester Courier and Lancashire General Advertiser
Manchester Guardian
Nottingham Evening Post
Portsmouth Evening News
Salford Weekly News
Sheffield Independent
Staffordshire Sentinel and Commercial and General Advertiser
The Times
The Times Literary Supplement
Urania
Western Daily Press

4. *Court Records*

These can include indictments that list an individual's name and address, depositions of evidence taken by the court, and transcripts of the trial proceedings. Where records are missing or restricted in any way (such as within a set rule for privacy), newspaper accounts can make up for this to a degree. Records for the coroner are kept separately.

5. *Prison Records*

    Will sometimes include photographs of the miscreant, past convictions, details of charge and sentence, whereabouts, trade, distinguishing marks and place of birth.

6. *Parliamentary Papers and Acts of Parliament*

    Acts of Parliament referred to in this book:

    1533: Buggery Act
    1836: Registration Act
    1840: Church Discipline Act
    1840: Vaccination Act (and 1853, 1867, 1898)
    1851: Common Lodging Houses Act
    1857: Matrimonial Causes Act
    1857: Obscene Publications Act
    1861: Offences Against the Person Act
    1870: Education Act
    1872: Licensing Act
    1875: Explosives Act
    1880: Education Act
    1882: Married Women's Property Act
    1885: Criminal Law Amendment Act
    1891: Slander of Women Act
    1898: Vagrancy Act
    1914: Defence of the Realm Act
    1921: Criminal Law Amendment Act
    1956: Sexual Offences Act

7. *Police Records*

    See also prison records: similar records may be available.

8. *Armed Forces Records*

    For those who served in the armed forces, especially after 1922, strictly limited access is available and usually only to next of kin. Prior to that, what records there are sometimes digitised where they have survived and may be available online.

9. *Oral History Sources*

- The Hall Carpenter Archives (HCA) has a large collection of interviews relating to same-sex experiences in Britain. The collection is based on a project begun in 1985. It also has a selection of archival sources dating from the beginning of the twentieth century. The collection is held at the London School of Economics.
- British Library Sound Archive: email: oralhistory@bl.uk. A search using the key word 'homosexual' brings up over 300 'hits', of which a high percentage seem to be interviews.

10. *Specialist Archives*

- The Women's Library Collection is housed in London and has useful content: http://www.lse.ac.uk/library/collections/featuredCollections/womensLibraryLSE.aspx
- The Lesbian and Gay News Media Archive: www.lagna.org enquiry@lagna.org.uk. Based in London, this is a vast collection of approximately 200,000 cuttings from all parts of the press relating to aspects of homosexual life from the 1930s onwards. It also houses a fair sized library of relevant titles.
- King's College Archive Centre, Cambridge: www.kings.cam.ac.uk/ archive-centre archivist@kings.cam.ac.uk. This archive holds the papers of Alan Turing.

11. *Magazines and Journals*

Will provide valuable contemporary views on family, culture and relationships. Some journals are digitised and available online, but normally a subscription is required for access. Check with county and national archive catalogues for holdings. The 'agony page' of a women's magazine can be very illuminating as to the advice given women who were questioning their sexuality or that of a family member.

12. *Wills and Probate Documents*

Possible insights into the relationships and inner circle of an individual. Prior to 1858, all wills are kept at local archives as they were proved in a church court; there is often an online catalogue you can search and perhaps even order online. After 1858, the probate service took over and wills can be searched for online in the Index to Wills 1858 onwards and copies ordered directly.

Location: local archives (pre 1858); Central Probate Registry post 1858.

13. *Divorce Records*

As we have seen in the main narrative, sometimes a homosexual relationship (male or female) was cited in divorce proceedings as grounds for divorce. You are much more likely to find divorces in your family history well into the twentieth century as they were almost impossible for ordinary working people to obtain earlier than that. A likely scenario for any person without the money to pay for legal proceedings was simply to part company with their spouse, and move elsewhere to set up a new life. A cross dressing or conventionally looking partnership may even have married again – bigamously – but this was very hard to track down prior to the twentieth century and is often the reason family historians look in vain for the death registration of a previous spouse which cannot be found. The answer is because your ancestor has told the registrar or clergyman, with a completely straight face, that they are widowed when they are not!

Location: For more recent records, where they have survived, apply to the court in the first instance. Divorces involving a homosexual relationship may have been featured in the local newspaper, so check these too.

14. *Health and Welfare Records*

Because homosexuality was seen as an illness for much of the nineteenth and twentieth centuries, this has generated records in the health care agencies. At the National Archives, records collections MH (Ministry of Health), HO (Home Office) and PCOM (Medical Research Council) may have useful material in them.

Local archives may have records relating to those committed to lunatic asylums and mental hospitals (as they were later known) because of their sexuality. Expect records concerning individual patients to be closed for one hundred years due to protection of privacy. National

Health Service general practitioner records for a patient are destroyed ten years after the patient's death and would be confidential in any case. See also prison records.

Location: hospital records will be at the county archive, although occasionally they will be at the hospital where it still exists. Records for former mental health institutions and workhouse infirmaries will be at the county archives.

15. *Records at the National Archives:*

National Archives

(The following information is a precis of advice from a National Archives research guide to LGBT research)

Armed forces: search on the National Archives website (see website list) using these department codes: ADM, WO, AIR and DEFE to look for records about relevant files relating to attitudes within the armed forces and in the War Office to homosexuality. These files may include records relating to people who were prosecuted, court martialled or discharged for sexual offences.

Censorship: the online catalogue can be used to find papers relating to prosecutions and censorship carried out under the Obscenity laws. Records from the following departments may be of use: Home Office (HO), Lord Chancellor's Office (LCO), Central Criminal Court (CRIM), and Director of Public Prosecutions (DPP).

Correspondence and papers from the Prime Minister's Office: for the period covering the Wolfenden Committee, see PREM 11 and PREM 13.

Papers from the Committee on Homosexual Offences and Prostitution (the Wolfenden Committee), 1954–1957: HO 345 and HO 291.

16. *Mass Observation*

In 1937, a social survey was begun which has become a key source of information about the opinions and lifestyles of a wide variety of people through their diaries, and through surveys conducted by the study. The aim of 'Mass Obs' as it became known was to find out what people thought about the widest possible spectrum of issues, one of which was homosexuality. The archive is based at Sussex University but is best learned about via the website: www. massobs.org.uk.

A Note About Online Networking

Many family and social historians now use a variety of online networking techniques to contact other researchers who have complementary interests to theirs. History forums, messaging via subscription-based family history research websites (see list of websites, below), and social media such as Facebook can provide a quick and seemingly easy way to contact people and share information and ideas. However, some simple guidelines can help make the experience of online networking safe and pleasurable.

When registering for a history forum, use an online username rather than your own, and never reveal your address, phone number, or any financial details, to anyone. If you contact someone in your extended family – say, a second or third cousin you do not know personally – about a relative you believe was homosexual or had some form of same-sex relationship, do be aware that not everyone will be as accepting of such relationships as you are. Just because someone is related to you at some level does not mean that they have had the same cultural, religious or educational influences as you, and there are many individuals, for example, who may still feel shame about having an illegitimacy in the family, let alone a homosexual relative. Discretion is particularly advised if the person you are enquiring about is recently deceased or belongs to a generation not that far removed from your contact. You get more information and goodwill by treading softly and treating your contacts with sensitivity.

Bibliography

Fiction with Same-sex Themes, First Published 1700–1957

Cleland, John: *Memoirs of a Woman of Pleasure*. (London, G. Fenton, 1749)

Fielding, Henry: *The Female Husband*. (London, M. Cooper, 1746)

Fitzroy, A.T.: *Despised and Rejected*. (London, C.W. Daniel, 1918)

Forster, Edward Morgan: *Maurice*. (written 1913; published for the first time London, Edward Arnold, 1971)

Hall, Radclyffe: *Miss Ogilvy Finds Herself*. (London, William Heinemann, 1934)

Hall, Radclyffe: *The Unlit Lamp*. (London,Cassell, 1924)

Hall, Radclyffe: *The Well of Loneliness*. (London, Jonathan Cape, 1928)

Lehmann, Rosamond: *Dusty Answer*. (London, Chatto and Windus, 1928)

Mackenzie, Compton: *Extraordinary Women*. (London, Martin Secker, 1928)

Oxenham, E.J. *The Abbey Girls Win Through*. (London, Collins, 1928)

Wilde, Oscar: *De Profundis*. (New York G P Putnam, 1905)

Wilde, Oscar: *The Picture of Dorian Gray*. (first book edition, Ward, Lock and Co, London, 1891)

Woolf, Virginia: *Orlando*. (London, Hogarth Press, 1928)

Non Fiction contemporary to the period 1700–1957

Anonymous (1749). *Satan's Harvest Home: or the Present State of Whorecraft, Adultery, Fornication, Procuring, Pimping, Sodomy, And the Game of Flatts, (Illustrated by an Authentick and Entertaining Story) And other Satanic Works, daily propagated in this good Protestant Kingdom*. (London, printed for the editor, and sold at the Change, St Paul's, Fleet Street, by Dod; Lewis; Exeter Change, and in the Court of Requests; Jackson, Jolliffe, Dodsley, Brindley, Steidel, Shropshire, Chappel, Hildyard, at York; Leak, at Bath; and at the snuff shop in Cecil Court, St. Martin's Lane, 1749)

BIBLIOGRAPHY

Charke, Charlotte: *A Narrative of the Life of Mrs Charlotte Charke, Youngest Daughter of Colley Cibber, Written by Herself.* (London, W. Reeve, 1755)

Freud, Sigmund: *Three Essays on the Theory of Sexuality.* (Leipzig and Vienna, Franz Deuticke, 1905; translated into English by A.A. Brill, 1910)

Hesnard, Angelo Louis Marie: *Strange Lust: the psychology of homosexuality.* (English translation by J C Summers, United States, American Ethnological Press, 1933)

Kinsey, Alfred C. et al.: *Sexual Behaviour in the Human Male.* (Philadelphia, Saunders, 1948)

Kinsey, Alfred C. et al.: *Sexual Behaviour in the Human Female.* (Philadelphia, Saunders, 1953)

Laycock,Thomas: *A Treatise on the Nervous Disorders of Women.* (London, Longman, 1840)

McQueen-Pope, W.: *Ivor: the story of an achievement.* (London, W.H. Allen, 1951)

Magian, A.C.: *Sex Problems in Women.* (London, Heinemann, 1922)

Stopes, Marie Carmichael: *A Journal From Japan: a daily record of life as seen by a scientist.* (London, Blackie, 1910)

Stopes, Marie Carmichael: *Enduring Passion; Further New Contributions to the Solution of Sex Difficulties Being the Continuation of Married Love.* (London, Hogarth Press, 1923)

Symonds, John Addington: *A Problem in Greek Ethics: Being an Inquiry into the Phenomenon of Sexual Inversion Addressed Especially to Medical Psychologists and Jurists.* (London, privately printed second edition, 1901)

Ward, Edward 'Ned': *The London Spy.* (London, 1703)

Wildeblood, Peter: *Against the Law.* (London, Harmondsworth, 1955)

Wolfenden, Sir John: *The Report of the Departmental Committee on Homosexual Offences and Prostitution ("The Wolfenden Report").* (London, HM Government, 1957)

Published Sources later than the period covered

Non Fiction

Anon: *Source Guide for the History of Manchester's Lesbian, Gay, Bisexual and Transgender Community.* (Manchester, 2011 edition)

Aldrich, Robert: *Gay Life and Culture: a world history.* (London, Thames and Hudson, 2006)

Bell, Barbara: *Just Take Your Frock Off: a lesbian life.* (Brighton, Ourstory Books, 1999)

Boughner, Terry: *Out of All Time: a gay and lesbian history.* (Alyson Publications, Boston, 1988)

Braun, Walter: *Lesbian Love: women in love throughout the ages.* (London, Senate, 1966)

Castle, Terry (editor): *The Literature of Lesbianism: an historical anthology from Ariosto to Stonewall.* (New York, Columbia University Press, 2003)

Castle, Terry: *Noel Coward and Radclyffe Hall: Kindred Spirits.* (New York, Colombia University Press, 1996)

Copeland, B. Jack: *Turing: pioneer of the information age.* (London, Oxford University Press, 2012)

DeSalvo, Louise and Leaska, Mitchell A.: *The Letters of Vita Sackville-West to Virginia Woolf.* (London, Hutchinson, 1984)

Donoghue, Emma: *Passions Between Women: British lesbian culture 1668–1801.* (London, Scarlet Press, 1993)

Ellimen, Michael and Roll, Frederick: *The Pink Plaque Guide to London.* (London, GMP Publishers, 1986)

Ellman, Richard: *Oscar Wilde.* (London, Hamish Hamilton, 1987)

Findlater, Richard: *Lilian Baylis: the lady of the Old Vic.* (London, Allen Lane, 1975)

Glasgow, Joanne (editor): *The Love Letters of Radclyffe Hall.* (New York, New York University Press, 1997)

Haggerty, George: *Men in Love: masculinity and sexuality in the eighteenth century.* (New York, Columbia University Press, 1999)

Halberstam, Judith: *Female Masculinity.* (Durham, Duke University Press, 1998)

Jennings, Rebecca: *A Lesbian History of Britain: love and sex between women since 1500.* (Oxford, Greenwood World Publishing, 2007)

Jivani, Alkarim: *It's Not Unusual: a history of lesbian and gay Britain in the twentieth century.* (London, Michael O'Mara Books by arrangement with the BBC, 1997)

LGBT Foundation: *Unlocking a Hidden History.* (Manchester, LGBT Foundation, 2013 edition)

Leaska, Mitchell A and Phillips, John: *Violet to Vita: the letters of Violet Trefusis to Vita Sackville-West.* (London, Mandarin, 1990)

Lesbian History Group: *Not a Passing Phase: reclaiming lesbians in history, 1840–1985.* (London, The Women's Press, 1989)

BIBLIOGRAPHY

Lewis, Gifford: *Eva Gore-Booth and Esther Roper: a biography.* (London, Pandora, 1988)

Liddington, Jill: *Female Fortune: land, gender and authority; the Anne Lister diaries and other writings, 1833–36.* (London, Rivers Oram Press, 1998)

McLaren, Angus: *Sexual Blackmail: a modern history.* (Harvard, Harvard University Press, 2002)

Magee, Bryan: *One in Twenty: a study of homosexuality in men and women.* (London, Secker and Warburg, 1966)

Marcus, Sharon: *Between Women: friendship, desire and marriage in Victorian England.* (Princeton, New Jersey, Princeton University Press, 2007)

Naphy, William: *Born to be Gay: a history of homosexuality.* (Stroud, Tempus Publishing, 2004)

National Archives, Archus Group: *LGBT History in TNA: list of documents.* (London, National Archives, 2014)

Newton, Esther: *The Mythic Mannish Lesbian: Radclyffe Hall and the new woman.* (Chicago, Signs, Vol. 9 No. 4, Summer 1984, The Lesbian Issue, pp 557–575)

Nicolson, Nigel: *Portrait of a Marriage.* (London, Weidenfeld and Nicolson, 1973)

Oram, Alison: *Feminism, Androgyny and Love Between Women in Urania, 1916–1940.* (London, Media History, 7:1, 57–70, 2001)

Oram, Alison and Turnbull, Annmarie: *The Lesbian History Sourcebook: love and sex between women in Britain from 1780 to 1970.* (Routledge, London, 2001)

Payn, Graham and Morley, Sheridan: *The Noel Coward Diaries.* (London, Weidenfeld and Nicholson, 1982)

Rich, Adrienne: *Blood, Bread and Poetry: selected prose 1979–1985.* (New York, Norton, 1987)

Saslow, James: *Pictures and Passions: a history of homosexuality in the visual arts.* (London, Viking Penguin, 1999)

Simpson, Ruth: *From the Closet to the Courts: the lesbian transition.* (London, Penguin Books, 1977)

Sinfield, Alan: *The Wilde Century.* (London, Cassell, 1994)

Souhami, Diana: *The Trials of Radclyffe Hall.* (London, Virago Press, 1999)

Souhami, Diana: *Wild Girls: the love life of Natalie Barney and Romaine Brooks.* (London, Weidenfeld and Nicholson, 2004)

Stanley, Liz: *Romantic Friendship? Some issues in researching lesbian history and biography.* (London, Women's History Review, 1:2, 193–216, 03-08-2006)

Stevens, Hugh (editor): *The Cambridge Companion to Gay and Lesbian Writing.* (Cambridge, Cambridge University Press, 2011)

Storey, Neil R. and Housego, Molly: *Women in the First World War.* (Oxford, Shire Publications, 2010)

Summers, Claude J. (editor): *The Gay and Lesbian Literary Heritage.* (London edition, Bloomsbury, 1997)

Summers, Claude J. (editor): *The Queer Encyclopaedia of Film and Television.* (San Francisco, Cleis Press, 2005)

Wachman, Guy: *Lesbian Empire: radical crosswriting in the twenties.* (New Jersey, Rutgers University Press, 2001)

Whitbread, Helena (editor). *No Priest But Love: the journal of Anne Lister from 1824–1826.* (Otley, Smith Settle, 1992)

Websites

(see also websites mentioned in resources, above)

Subscription-based research websites: two examples are www.ancestry.co.uk and www.findmypast.co.uk. Popular sources for digitised census returns, and indexes to civil registration, wills, parish registers and newspapers. If you decide to subscribe to such a website, take your time to look at a wide variety before committing yourself to any.

www.britishnewspaperarchive.co.uk. A subscription website, which probably has the best selection of digitized British newspapers to search online. Alternatively, check if your local library card offers free online access to other newspaper archives.

www.lgbthistorymonth.org.uk. LGBT History Month is held every February and this website offers updates on activities connected with that. It also hosts an annual conference.

http://www.rictornorton.co.uk/eighteen/1721news.htm Norton, Rictor (Ed.), 'Newspaper Reports, 1720–1723,' Homosexuality in Eighteenth-Century England: A Sourcebook. 3 March 2004, updated 10 December 2014 and 24 July 2015. Also an excellent source of stories of same-sex relationships, drawn from a variety of sources.

Index